FITNESS FOR YOUR LIFE

You Can Do It

Richard Giesbrecht

authorHOUSE®

AuthorHouse™
1663 Liberty Drive
Bloomington, IN 47403
www.authorhouse.com
Phone: 1-800-839-8640

© 2010 Richard Giesbrecht. All rights reserved.

No part of this book may be reproduced, stored in a retrieval system, or transmitted by any means without the written permission of the author.

First published by AuthorHouse 5/3/2010

ISBN: 978-1-4490-9602-1 (e)
ISBN: 978-1-4490-9613-7 (sc)

Library of Congress Control Number: 2010903272

Printed in the United States of America
Bloomington, Indiana

This book is printed on acid-free paper.

CONTENTS

Preface ix
The Fitness Journey 1
Overview 5
Exercise Applications Used 9
Why Is Health And Fitness Important? 15
Personal Realities 19
Know Yourself Before You Exercise 23
What "Training Zone" Should You Use? 41
Full Body Exercise Format 47
Training Program Methodology 55
Exercise Preparation 61
Set Your Goals 65
Track Your Progress 67
When Should You Work Out? 71
How Often Should You Workout? 75
How Long Should Your Workout Be? 79
Proper Form Is Crucial 81
Hints For A Successful Program 87

- Training Exercises And Drills 91
1. Warm Up 95
2. Cardio Options.. 107
3. Resistance (Strength)Training................................... 111
   - A. Lower Body exercises 112
   - B. Upper Body exercises 128
   - C. Core & Back exercises...................................... 140
4. Plyometrics 161
5. Martial Arts For Strength & Cardio............................ 175
   - A. Fundamentals.. 177
   - B. Applying The Fundamentals 183
6. Stretching And Cool Down... 199
   - A. Lower Body... 202
   - B. Upper Body... 222
   - C. Abs, Back & Neck... 229
- Sample Programs.. 238
  - Sample "Full Body" Beginner Program 240
  - Sample "Full Body"Intermediate Program............... 242
  - Sample "Full Body" Advanced Program.................. 244
  - Sample "Shock Treatment/Fat Burner" Program 246
  - Sample "Pyramid – Full Body Cardio" Program...... 248
  - Sample "Circuit" Program 249
  - Sample "Interval" Program....................................... 250
  - Sample Running Drills 252
    - Simple Wind Sprints.. 253

- Mountain Climb 254
- Spot Run Challenge 255
- The Office Program – 10 Minute Health Break 256
- Create Your Own Program 257
- Healthy Eating Suggestions 263
- Conclusion 271
- Acknowledgements 273

PREFACE

My drive to create this book was simply to share what knowledge I have gained over the years that has helped me maintain an affordable, healthy and fit lifestyle. There is a tremendous amount of fitness information currently available in the marketplace. Most of this material tends to concentrate on one particular type of exercise or fitness area. The focus of this book is to assist you in developing your own program with the aid of numerous exercises and workout drills taken from a wide variety of fitness disciplines. Since nutrition is a significant part of maintaining a fit and healthy lifestyle, this guide also provides some nutritional ideas and suggestions.

There are many options and approaches that you can take to help improve your fitness. This guide is based on the premise that everyone is different and, as such, a successful fitness program is very personal and sometimes unique. To that end, it is my intent to provide you with a wide variety of options that I hope you will find challenging while maintaining your interest. If you are a frequent traveler, this guide will even help you develop your own fitness program that you can utilize while you are "on the road".

This book is really a "how to" guide that tries to keep physical fitness simple and understandable, but not overly technical, while still being informative. A Twitter Account is available **(www.Twitter.com/ForevrFit.com)** so that you may reach out for clarifications, or new ideas you may have, related to the exercises or drills that are available within this guide. I have purposely avoided lengthy detailed chapters on technical matters but chose to focus on the actual form and application of a variety of exercises. Some technical information has been provided to help give you a basic understanding of some of the important aspects related to physical fitness. This includes things like knowing your physical limitations and gaining an introductory appreciation of your heart and other muscles.

The book is designed to help you prepare for and maintain a physically fit lifestyle, or enhance your current fitness program, with the wide array of exercise and program options provided like martial arts and interval training. It also provides some guidance in performing a fitness assessment, setting personal goals and determining how to get the best out of a workout.

There are no weights or gadgets required! Everything in this book relies solely on your body weight - similar to what the Olympiads did for their training when the Games were first created. All of the information in this book can be applied to men or women and all ages. All you really need is your own personal commitment, ongoing dedication, time, and last but not least.....**effort!**

The unfortunate reality is that the vast majority of people who start a fitness program drop out within the first three months. Even more astonishing is that of those who do continue beyond three months, only a select few adopt some kind of health and fitness approach as a way of life.

I am confident that with the tools provided within this guide it will help you stay the course in terms of a healthy and fit lifestyle.

THE FITNESS JOURNEY

The road to good health is a long and winding journey that tests personal commitment. I've learned from my own journey that it is no different than pursuing a successful professional career. First, you need to determine your special area of interest. Then you need to do some research and educate yourself. This knowledge leads to the formulation of your personal vision. Once you have a vision, you need to establish the path you want to take to realize that vision. That path may include numerous activities that would need to be completed. And finally, once you have begun your journey, you need to stay the course.

Although it all sounds very straightforward, actually achieving success depends on your ability to adapt to changes in your personal circumstances, your environment, your physical body and even your emotional state. And last but not least, you have to commit to giving it your best effort!

Based on my life experience, I am firmly convinced that to remain competitive, both professionally and personally, requires a "**healthy mind and a healthy body**". The two absolutely complement one another.

The level of stress created within the business environment, especially these days, is challenging and can be taxing. If you are not in good physical condition you can get worn down to the point that you are unable to think clearly, unable to absorb information to make informed decisions or unable to sustain the long demanding work hours required.

Generally speaking, if you are healthy, you typically have a more positive personality, are more outgoing and realize more personal and professional success.

It is my hope that this guide will provide you with at least one truth that you can carry forward forever. "**Fitness is for Your Life**" and it is within your personal control. This guide is a tool that can help support your fulfillment of that endeavor.

I started the fitness journey 44 years ago and have changed my approach to overall health and fitness numerous times. I firmly believe that you can slow down the aging process by maintaining a strong health and fitness regimen. Since the body goes through tremendous changes during its life cycle, we need to continue to look at what we do to stay fit and be prepared to adapt our fitness routines accordingly so we can continue to challenge our bodies. Over the years, I have changed the types of activities I've participated in. I've routinely changed the types of workouts I have and I continue to change the types of exercises and drills used in my workouts. Furthermore, I continually look at different ways to improve my approach towards nutrition.

It is no surprise that the success associated with any fitness program is contingent upon a number of factors and one of those is nutrition. Although the focus of this guide is to provide guidance in terms of developing interesting and challenging fitness programs and drills, there are aspects of nutrition that are introduced.

Along with a high level of commitment, I would suggest that "**change**" is necessary for any successful health or fitness program. I have observed that success is typically enjoyed by those who adapt to change and also use change for their benefit. This will become more evident as you progress through this guide since the concept of change is applied throughout to help improve fitness.

I believe the benefits I have enjoyed through the **"fitness for my life"** approach which includes many of the exercises, drills and programs

I personally utilize can also help you. The overall approach, and concepts presented within this guide, is an affordable means to help promote individual fitness and health as a way of life. The majority of the exercises, drills and programs included can be done at any age, at any place, and performed throughout a lifetime. I would also suggest that this guide is a great companion for the business traveler who might have a hard time finding a gym or has a busy travel schedule (even a sample workout for The Office has been provided to show you how creative you can be in terms of applying this guide).

Fitness for Your Life does not require a fitness membership; space is not an issue; equipment is not necessary; and there is no need for a professional trainer (unless you choose to use one).

You can get a good start on your own by utilizing this book as your guide, using your own personal initiative and acquiring some light workout gear. Depending on the level of fitness you want to achieve, and your ongoing interest level, you may some day decide to invest in a fitness membership, trainer or equipment. If nothing else, when you cross that bridge, this book will have provided you with some fitness knowledge and experience so that you have greater confidence in taking those steps.

OVERVIEW

The framework for this guide follows 4 key principles; 1) maintain a full body balanced workout; 2) an effective workout can be done anywhere – space is not an issue; 3) it is for all ages and; 4) maintain variety, change and challenge. The guide is designed to help young adolescents, the busy traveling professional and the elderly without the need for gadgets, equipment, memberships or perhaps even trainers. Simply put, my goal is to help you achieve **"Fitness for Your Life"** by taking your own initiative and empowering you, while using my guide, to help focus your efforts to realize success.

Over 200 exercises and drills are included in this guide. They have been derived from various types of physical fitness concepts and mind body applications. They can be assembled in many different ways to provide a full body workout while allowing for program variety. They cover most parts of the body involving cardiovascular development, strength and muscular development and include help with improving flexibility, balance, coordination, agility and speed.

The guide can be used by the novice and the fitness fanatic. It is designed to help you get started with a fitness program, even if you do not have prior experience, while challenging those that are more seasoned in terms of a fitness discipline.

For those of you who find that exercise can be boring, this guide will help overcome some of those feelings by offering numerous exercise options, training applications and program designs to help create and maintain variety while still challenging the body. For those of you that already enjoy an exercise regimen, I am confident the guide will help provide a new and challenging experience.

Some guidance will be provided in terms of helping you understand your current level of health and fitness. However, you should always consider advice from your doctor before starting any type of fitness program. Once you have established your starting point, this guide will provide the information and advice to help you every step of the way towards a healthier and fit lifestyle. For those of you that are relatively new to exercising, some suggestions are provided to help you get the best out of your body for an effective workout. This also includes some ideas involving nutrition.

Sample programs are also included to get you started so that you can gain experience with the numerous exercises and drills made available. Once you feel comfortable with the exercises and sample programs, this guide can also help you create your own unique and challenging personal programs.

In terms of creating your own program, the guide is designed to help you with the following:

1. Preparing you for the fitness challenge, mentally and physically, if you are not already involved with fitness;

2. Assisting you with the creation of personal goals and monitoring progress for continuous improvement;

3. Developing a full body exercise program format that includes a warm up, cardio, strength, flexibility and a cool down – and even coordination, agility, speed and balance;

4. Defining your area of focus such as the upper body, the lower body and your core;

5. Maintaining variety so that your body is always challenged while keeping the program interesting for you and;

6. Helping you to explore and be creative so that you can develop your own exercises and programs.

A significant number of exercises are included in this guide that will help you get healthier and improve your fitness. The only thing this book does not provide is your own will power and personal commitment to stay with it. Remember, you do not have to be a seasoned or highly paid athlete to get fit while maintaining a healthy appearance and lifestyle. You really are in control of your own destiny.

EXERCISE APPLICATIONS USED

The exercises and drills included within this guide have been derived from various types of physical fitness applications and mind/body approaches culminating from years of teaching, training and personal experience. They include calisthenics, plyometrics, aerobics, isotonics, isometrics, yoga and martial arts to name a few.

You will find that the exercises and drills included are "well rounded" and geared towards a full body fitness approach because they address the key aspects of physical fitness conditioning: warm ups, resistance (strength) training, cardiovascular conditioning, speed, agility, quickness, flexibility, coordination, balance and cool down.

Since proper form is essential for making positive gains, a very specific procedure accompanies each exercise, along with pictures, to show how they should be performed.

As you become familiar with the contents of this guide, and become more experienced with the exercises and programs included, you will find that you can modify them to continually challenge your body and maintain your interest. The physical fitness applications utilized in this guide are also described in detail so that you will understand and appreciate the context of the exercises.

CALISTHENIC EXERCISES

Calisthenics is Greek in origin and is made from the words kalos (beautiful) and sthenos (strength). These types of exercises are bodyweight exercises that come from gymnastics concepts. Typically, they do not require any equipment and are convenient to do. Calisthenics are utilized to help improve overall fitness and strength while promoting grace in physical movements of the body. A couple of examples include pushups and jumping jacks. On their own, they are a great way to build and tone muscle. When they are combined with other movements they are tremendous for enhancing endurance, strength and burning fat. For example, you might perform pushups to place focus on your chest development. Between push up sets, you may chose to perform some jumping jacks as they place less focus on your chest and more on your legs. Since the focus is shifted to the legs from the upper body, they provide "active rest" while continuing to burn calories. We'll cover this in more detail later on in the guide.

PLYOMETRIC EXERCISES

Even though plyometric exercises typically find their place in training programs related to numerous types of sports, like hockey, they can be very effective for improving your overall fitness level. Plyometrics are a type of high intensity exercise that typically involves some form of jumping or hopping movements. The key principle behind plyometrics is the stretching and shortening cycle of the muscles involved in the exercise. Because of this movement, the muscles become more efficient over time and store more elastic energy. This helps to provide powerful, explosive muscle response while enhancing the intensity of a workout.

Although there are varying opinions on the use of plyometrics for training purposes, The American Council on Fitness "recommends using plyometric exercises provided they are done properly". These types of exercises have a tendency to significantly increase caloric burn and include ones like the squat jump. This will be addressed in more detail in a later chapter involving differing types of plyometric exercises.

CARDIOVASCULAR EXERCISES

This type of exercise is typically an activity or type of movement that is sustained for a period of time, usually for a minimum of 20-30 minutes, which helps develop cardio-respiratory endurance. These exercises can improve circulatory and respiratory efficiency and lung capacity. They include activities like swimming, aerobics and running. This type of training is an essential component of any fitness program in terms of enhancing aerobic and anaerobic capacity. In simple terms, it can help improve your endurance and stamina so that you can go longer and further before "running out of steam".

Cardiovascular exercise, or fitness, also has other benefits. As your aerobic and anaerobic capacity increases, your general metabolism, along with your muscle metabolism, increases while your flow of blood improves. Indirectly, this will help improve your strength and flexibility over time.

Because of the nature of this type of exercise or activity, the larger muscles (legs) and joints (hips) are the ones that become the focus. These types of exercises work very well in terms of promoting leanness, and reducing your BMI (Body Mass Index), which will be addressed later.

ISOTONIC EXERCISES

There are two types of isotonic exercises. One is called concentric and the other is eccentric. A concentric movement means that the external force being placed on the muscle is less than the actual force that the muscle is generating. The squat is an example of a concentric exercise because the quad muscle becomes shorter as the leg is extended from the squat position. Eccentric movement is the opposite of a concentric one. As the muscle gains more tension it lengthens. These types of exercise movements are not as common. Jumping or going down stairs are eccentric type movements that will be included in some of the exercises in this guide. Typically, isotonic types of exercises help improve muscle tone and the functionality of joints.

ISOMETRIC EXERCISES

This type of exercise involves a static positioning of the muscle since it does not change and is held for the duration chosen to perform the exercise. Movement of the muscle is isometric in nature. An example of an isometric exercise is the plank, or the prone position, that is used to work the abs and lower back.

YOGA

Yoga is an approach to fitness that is based on an ancient form of physical movement that helps to promote balance, flexibility, strength and relaxation through various poses and breathing techniques. I have found there are some similarities in terms of martial arts applications that are of tremendous benefit in terms of overall physical fitness. Yoga strives to help create an inner peace through a combination of movements and controlled, but relaxing, breathing techniques. There are numerous stretching techniques that have been derived from Yoga in this book. For these reasons, you will find that the philosophy is incorporated into the cool down aspects of the workouts prescribed. This has been done specifically to ensure that the hard work and efforts expended during a full body workout are truly enjoyed after the experience.

MARTIAL ARTS

A few fundamentals of Martial Arts are included in this guide to add variety and challenge from a physical fitness perspective. Although they are limited, they do provide the basis for numerous martial arts defense strategies that also have physical fitness attributes as well.

Martial Arts is a wonderful philosophy that can help improve self-confidence, self-esteem and even help you find personal spirituality. Your spirituality can be invaluable in terms of helping stay the "health and fitness" course by assisting with overcoming physical and mental limitations. It can teach you to have faith in yourself, to never quit and always challenge yourself. It can also help teach self discipline, mentally and/or physically, when dealing with training in isolation.

The specific techniques introduced stem from an Oriental form of self-defense called Wado Kai. This particular style is a culmination of other martial arts forms that involve kick boxing, kung fu and tae kwon do. This is an ideal style to assist with fitness training because it lends itself to improving leanness (through an enhanced caloric burn), cardiovascular and muscular development, strength, speed and coordination. For the purpose of this guide, the primary focus will be on blocking, punching and kicking techniques. However, there are various other techniques that will be utilized (consistent with Yoga) to assist with the Cool Down component of the workout such as breathing, stretching and simple relaxation.

WHY IS HEALTH AND FITNESS IMPORTANT?

There are numerous reasons for improving and maintaining your fitness level and overall health. They may be medical, personal, for your family or it may even be a requirement of your employer. From a personal perspective, you may simply want a different way of life, to provide a good example for your family or simply to do it for enjoyment.

Over time, exercise can actually become a necessity, as it has for me. Something is missing if I skip a session. In that regard, fitness can become a positive addiction. Regardless of the reason, it is my strong opinion that any effort to improve personal health and fitness is the right direction to take.

Some other reasons for improving your health and fitness level might include the following:

Confidence and Self-Esteem – positive physical conditioning can improve the way you feel about yourself, your abilities, your self-worth and even how attractive you feel. It can even have a positive impact on your personal and professional success simply due to your outlook on things.

Osteoporosis – improved fitness levels help increase muscle mass and provide greater strength. This adds density to the bones making them stronger and reduces the risk of osteoporosis.

Family – typically it is easier to stay fit and remain active as a family rather than trying to do it on your own. I have also found from my own training experiences that people generally find it more challenging to maintain and prepare different meals for individual family members. I might also add that it is easier for children, and even more enjoyable for them to develop healthy lifestyles, if they see their parents leading by example.

Aging – by the age of 60, we generally loose about one third of our muscle tissue and tend to increase body fat. After the age of 50, we typically loose about 10% of our strength every 10 years. In my opinion, staying fit is a great way to fight off the aging process, especially if the program includes the essential "stretching" ingredient. Stretching for enhanced flexibility also enhances muscular and cardiovascular development.

Leanness – healthier bodies have greater muscle mass and a higher metabolism. As a result, they become more efficient in terms of burning calories. Even though a fit person may weigh more, they may be leaner because muscle weighs more than fat and they will burn more calories to help maintain the muscle.

Stress – being physically fit can help make it easier to relax and shed the tensions created by work or personal circumstances. A good workout, even just a good brisk walk, can help combat tension and get you through difficult periods.

Reduced Healthcare Costs – there is little doubt that the Baby Boomers (Zoomers) are going to place an increased burden on the cost of providing healthcare. Those who maintain a fit and healthy lifestyle through their advancing years will not need to rely on Health Care as much as those in less healthier circumstances. The healthier crowd will typically be able to save money for more pleasurable things over the long term.

Reduced Risk of Injury - higher levels of fitness and flexibility will typically help reduce the risk of injury. All too often, individuals who do nothing for extended periods find that weekends and special occasions require physical exertion that their body is not prepared for (I call them "weekend warriors"). While we may think our bodies will respond like they did when we were younger, they often don't. This can result in sore or hurt muscles, or even muscles that may not respond when called upon.

Cross Training – maintaining an exercise program, of any type, helps to enhance athletic sports performance. Participating in a variety of physically demanding and challenging activities provides cross training benefits because it adds variety and ongoing challenges for the body.

Healthy Mind – I truly believe that a healthy body and a healthy mind go hand in hand. Typically, improved levels of fitness can make you more alert and help you think more clearly, make better decisions and perform better in school or at work (I firmly believe this is what got me through University). The mind stays fresh and can absorb more.

Energy & Endurance – since a fit body has increased muscle mass, it can do more with less effort even though it burns more calories. This certainly helps to improve overall individual pleasure, like playing sports or taking care of work around the yard, because of reduced fatigue.

Reduced Blood Pressure - a healthier body, healthier heart and healthier circulatory system all go hand-in-hand with controlling blood pressure and providing a more enjoyable and fulfilling lifestyle.

Although the above list is not a comprehensive one, it does help us understand why we exercise to maintain a healthier lifestyle.

PERSONAL REALITIES

Before you begin your fitness journey, you should try to understand your personal attributes as they will influence your approach and perhaps even the success you achieve. Your personal attributes consist of the tangible and intangible realities that make each of us unique human beings. The intangibles include things like your attitude, your commitment and the effort you put forth. The tangibles include those characteristics you are born with and involve your body composition (physique) and your heart (due to its importance, there are dedicated sections on the heart in future chapters). Once we understand the attributes that we have been blessed with, it makes it easier for us to use them for our benefit.

YOUR ATTITUDE

Try to keep in mind that people with a positive attitude tend to be happier and mentally stronger. They try to find ways to accomplish their professional and personal goals no matter what roadblocks they are faced with. I sometimes feel this might be something you are born with but, if you are not, I truly believe that you can develop it within yourself. A physically strong body and healthy lifestyle will provide greater confidence, self-esteem and reduce the shyness or insecurity you may be feeling. It can help you feel confident enough to take on more challenges and bring you the success you deserve from your efforts.

YOUR EFFORT, COMMITMENT AND DEDICATION

Personal effort, commitment and dedication over time are some of the key ingredients that can help you become successful. If you put forth a strong effort (sweating is not bad) while remaining committed and dedicated to your fitness program, I am confident you will see positive results and achieve your goals.

On occasion, I have come to observe some interesting approaches that people have adopted for their exercise regimen. They caught my attention, due to their apparent lack of success, and for this reason I would like to share them with you as something to avoid. I took note of a few individuals that looked like they were trying the "buddy system" of working out. This is a great approach to encourage one another, especially if you are just starting out. After witnessing many of their workout sessions over a period of weeks (each session being anywhere from 45-90 minutes in duration), I noticed they did not sweat, were not flushed in the face and did not show any signs of physically challenging themselves. What is interesting is that these individuals could not understand why they were not seeing any progress. This reinforces that you can be highly dedicated and committed to your program, however, if you are lacking key pieces of information that may need to be applied, your results may be limited.

Although I do not profess to know their specific individual circumstances, it seems to me these individuals were not making progress because they were exercising at a rate well below their personal Training Heart Rate Zone. Essentially, they had not even moved out of the "warm up stage" of a workout. As such, their bodies were not challenged to work and their hearts did not strive for, or even reach, any cardiovascular gains. This reinforces that you can be highly dedicated and committed to your program, however, if you are lacking key pieces of information that may need to be applied, your results may be limited.

I bring this up just in case you find yourself in a similar situation. It can be a simple correction once you understand the potential issue. My suggestion is that you consider reviewing your Target Heart Rate Training Zone. We will cover this in a later section so that you can gain an appreciation of where you may want to be in this regard.

You may also want to consult a certified trainer and/or your physician if you are not sure if your assessment is correct for your particular circumstance.

Here is another common situation. Let's say one of your goals is to lose weight. That being the case, you should pay attention to the total calories you need to burn. Typically, .45 kilograms (one pound) of stored fat is equal to 3500 stored calories (keep in mind heavier people will burn more calories than lighter people when performing the same activity). That means if you eat 500 more calories each day than your body uses to function, exercise or perform various activities, you would gain .45 kilograms in one week. Since there are differing opinions on the relationship between caloric burn and weight gain, I suggest this serve as a guide only. The point that I want to make is that there seems to be a direct relationship between effort and intensity of a workout and the number of calories burned and weight lost.

If we go back to our earlier scenario involving the frustrated individuals, only two weeks after a couple of them increased their Training Heart Rate Zone, they noticed considerable improvement. One person lost 2 kg (approx. 4 pounds) and the other actually reduced their waistline by almost 25mm (one inch). Obviously these types of results will vary by person.

Although the above are small examples, they do show that understanding your body and how it functions can help you get the results you want. Furthermore, the effort you expend is important and simply going through the motions typically does not help realize success.

One test of commitment and dedication involves maintaining your workout schedule. It is very easy to pass on a workout when you have a busy schedule that consumes your day. Unfortunately, it is not uncommon for people to miss one workout, then another and another, and before you know it, months have passed by and another person has stopped traveling the road to improved health and fitness.

Even if you try to complete a small part of your program, instead of nothing at all, it will help to keep you engaged. Although this may seem trivial, my past experience has shown this to be quite important. This simple approach will not only help to maintain your focus and commitment but it can even provide a refreshing 5 minute break during a stressful day (close your office door and do a few push ups or sit ups). You might also be surprised how this opens the mind to address your challenges at work or school. Once you overcome these temptations to put off a workout you are well on your way to maintaining **"Fitness for Your Life"**.

YOUR PHYSIQUE

It is important to recognize that not everyone is naturally fit, a gifted athlete, or even born looking like a Greek God. Few people are born with perfect body composition. As frustrating as it may be, there are those that don't need to watch what they eat, and don't ever exercise, yet they look physically toned and well proportioned. Their body composition just does not seem to change no matter what they do or don't do to it.

Even if you are not an athlete, it does not mean you cannot be athletic or stay in reasonably good physical condition. What is important is that you feel good about yourself. In simple terms, do what you can to the best of your ability with what you naturally have been blessed with. Sometimes that means that some individuals will have more natural ability than others. It may also mean that some individuals may have to work harder to deal with and overcome personal obstacles that get in the way. It does not mean you cannot be successful and achieve the personal and professional goals you set for yourself. Life is all about overcoming and adapting.

KNOW YOURSELF BEFORE YOU EXERCISE

In the previous chapter you were introduced to some of the tangible and intangible personal attributes you bring to the table. Before you begin to exercise, you should determine if you have any types of issues, such as physical limitations, that may prevent you from doing certain things associated with a fitness program. If you do not know your starting point, it can make it challenging to identify your fitness direction, your personal goals and even any progress you want to make. You should consult with a family physician to understand your present health status and your family health history.

Once you have your doctor's blessing, and assuming your doctor has not already done so for you, I suggest you get to know a few other important things about yourself before starting your fitness program. Some of the things you might want to try and understand include your current lifestyle in terms of health and fitness level, your body composition, your flexibility, and your nutritional habits. These are areas where a professional trainer may be able to offer some assistance. However, if you have limited resources available to you, you can conduct your own cursory review to gain some appreciation of the parameters you are working within.

I have included some thoughts within this guide to help you with this investigation, however please note that they should not replace any advice you receive from a physician or a trainer. If nothing else, perhaps the information can assist you with any discussions you have with a professional so you are more informed and prepared with some good questions to ask.

HEALTH AND FITNESS REVIEW

Health and fitness reviews or evaluations complement fitness training because they help provide you with an indication of your current health status, including important aspects such as your Blood Pressure and your Heart, while isolating significant injuries or risks that might affect your ability to exercise. This is also why input from your doctor is critical.

It is important to keep track of your blood pressure. Normal Blood Pressure is 120mmHg/80mmHg. The mmHg means millimeters of mercury when your measurement is taken by your doctor. The 120mmHg is the systolic pressure or the amount of pressure created by the heart as it contracts on the walls of the arteries. The 80mmHg is the diastolic pressure, or the pressure on the walls of the arteries, from the heart relaxing and then filling up again with blood.

Obviously your heart is crucial and it is essential that you understand it. When you challenge your body you place degrees of work or exertion on your heart. The heart is not only an organ but a muscle that needs a workout too in order to help stay in good operating condition.

Since everyone is different, it is important to know your heart and its capacity or ability to undertake a rigorous workout. A physician is in the best position to assess your heart. Regardless, this section is intended to help provide some general guidance and information on the topic.

If your heart is not used to physical exertion, it may not be able to handle as much work as it could. Typically over time, with improved conditioning, it should have enhanced capacity. Keep in mind that the heart rate usually slows down as it becomes more accustomed to exercise while its capacity reduces with age. This reality reinforces the need to continually change the manner and approach in the way you exercise for personal benefit.

To gain a greater appreciation of your heart and how it reacts to exercise, you should first try to understand your Resting Heart Rate, your Maximum Heart Rate and your Training Heart Rate Zone. This information will provide you with essential data that can help you to get the best out of your workout, in terms of intensity level, without getting hurt. Due to the their importance during physical exertion, these differing heart rates will be addressed in much more detail in a future chapter dedicated to determining your training intensity level.

The fitness review will also help give you a greater appreciation or understanding of your body composition, muscular strength and endurance, your cardiovascular capacity and your flexibility. This important information will provide the foundation to create an exercise program that is specific to your needs and based on your current capabilities.

Another benefit of the fitness review is that it will assist you in the development of your personal fitness goals. It will provide you with your starting point so that you know where you are coming from and how well you are progressing. This information is also useful to help you determine when and if you need to fine tune your program to further your personal goals.

The following are some suggested questions that you could ask yourself, your physician or a trainer to gain an understanding of your personal physical fitness level:

1. Considering my age, am I in good physical condition?

2. Do I look good physically?

3. Do I have sufficient energy on a daily basis to work out?

4. Can I participate in activities using a moderate amount of effort?

5. Can I move around with minimal pain or limitation of movement in my legs, arms or back?

6. Can I handle continuous periods of cardiovascular activity?

7. Do I perform stretching and flexibility exercises on a regular basis?

There are numerous tools available through the internet that can also help provide additional information and assistance on this topic.

REVIEW YOUR MUSCLE AND ENDURANCE STRENGTH

There are different types of strength including emotional, spiritual and physical. Although all of them are essential for maintaining your personal well being, this guide will focus on the physical aspects including muscle strength and endurance. It is worth noting that some studies suggest that any improvements you realize in your physique correlate with developments you realize emotionally and spiritually too.

Basically, your muscles provide you with the strength you need to move your bones so that you can perform physically demanding day to day activities and functions. Muscle endurance, on the other hand, involves the capacity of the muscle to exert effort, or perform a particular activity, for an extended period of time.

Over the years, I have used a few fairly simple and straightforward exercises to help determine the muscle strength and endurance of individuals. The first one involves the "perfect form" push up (to be explained later). Other exercises involve the traditional push up, the typical sit up and the front lunge. These exercises are covered in detail in a later chapter and you may want to skip ahead to see their respective "forms" so that you can accurately conduct a simple test of your strength now.

To test yourself, I would suggest you attempt as many of these three exercises ensuring you follow proper form: standard push ups (on your hands and your knees, or toes); standard sit ups; and front lunges.

Although these exercises may seem easy, once perfect form is applied, they become much more challenging. To put things in perspective, a beginner might be challenged with 2 perfect form push ups while someone more fit may be able to complete 5-10.

This simple test, described above, will help determine your baseline fitness level prior to starting your training program, so you can track your improvement.

CARDIOVASCULAR REVIEW

Earlier it was noted that cardiovascular fitness is an important aspect of any fitness program. There are a number of approaches that can be taken to measure cardiovascular fitness. One approach is to select a type of cardiovascular drill, for example spot running, and try to perform it for as long as you can while maintaining proper form and the training heart rate zone prescribed by your doctor.

Another measure is your recovery time. This is simply how quickly you can recover from a high intensity workout or activity, and return to normal levels, in terms of heart beats per minute. Upon completion of a workout, take a measure of your heart beats per minute. The amount of time it takes you to return to your normal heart rate is one indication of cardiovascular fitness level. The shorter the recovery time the greater the cardiovascular fitness level (although this does vary by person, you can use it as an indicator of your progress).

You can also use your Resting Heart Rate as an indicator of your cardiovascular fitness. It is simply your heart rate when you first wake up in the morning. It will be addressed in the next chapter that involves calculating your heart rate zone for training purposes.

UNDERSTAND YOUR BODY COMPOSITION

In terms of physical fitness, and according to Wikipedia, "body composition is used to describe the percentage of fat, bone and muscle in human bodies". Since muscular tissue takes up less space in our body than fat tissue, our body composition, as well as our weight, determines leanness. For these reasons, two people that have the same height and weight can actually look very different from one another.

Your body composition is a measure of the difference between fat mass and fat-free mass (muscles, bones and internal organs). The ideal means for measuring body composition is hydrostatic weighing. This is an approach where your body is actually placed underwater and your normal body weight is compared to your underwater weight.

The Body Mass Indicator, or index (BMI), is a very common approach for measuring fat mass. BMI is an estimate of body composition that considers weight and height. A normal BMI ranges from 19 to 25 but keep in mind your BMI may not be the most accurate measurement for determining your health and fitness level.

To calculate your own BMI, take your weight and divide it by your height squared. The BMI for a person 1.83 meters (6 feet) tall and weighing 85 kg (189 pounds) would be as follows;

$$BMI = \frac{Weight\ (kg)}{Height\ (squared)}$$

$$BMI = \frac{85}{1.83 \times 1.83} = 25.37$$

NOTE: 1 kg = 2.22 pounds

1 meter = 39.37 inches

If you are concerned about your personal BMI, you should have a discussion with your family physician as individual circumstances can impact results.

Although BMI should be considered when undertaking a personal fitness review, it should be used only as another piece of information and not the only data to rely on in terms of determining your level of health. With respect to children or adolescents, BMI information should not be used for measuring progress or improvement because the growth and changes in their body composition make the data unreliable.

Also keep in mind that muscle weighs more than fat. As such, when you gain muscle and loose fat you may not necessarily see a significant reduction in weight loss. Instead, what you may start to notice is a shifting of body proportion and shape due to toning. A helpful approach to monitor progress in this regard involves taking measurements at key points on the body and checking those periodically for muscle gain or fat loss. This will also vary depending on your individual circumstances.

There are some key areas of your body to measure, PRIOR to starting your program and for monitoring purposes, such as:

1. Weight _____

2. Chest _____

3. Waist _____

4. Arm _____
   (elbow 90 degrees & measure widest point)

5. Thigh (uppermost area) _____

6. Hip (at the hip bone) _____

7. Buttocks _____
   (the widest point & feet together)

8. Calf (at the widest point) _____

The above measurements should be reviewed on a periodic basis. Monitoring them will help keep track of your progress and assist with modifications and focus of your individual exercise program. Weekly checks may be too frequent to notice change. However, monthly reviews typically tend to show more noticeable differences which you can then use to assess and determine your next steps.

WHAT IS YOUR FLEXIBILITY OR RANGE OF MOTION (ROM)

Your flexibility is an important element of your fitness program. Flexibility is essentially your ability to move a joint through a range of motion (ROM). Different people have differing levels of flexibility, or ROM, and women typically are more flexible than men because they have less muscle mass. Muscle mass has a tendency to limit joint movement.

Improved flexibility will help you to perform even routine daily activities such as cleaning the house and cutting the grass. Within this guide we will incorporate two of the more common types of stretching to assist with improving flexibility. The first and more traditional type is Static Stretching and the other is Dynamic Stretching.

Static stretching essentially involves focusing on a certain joint, like the knee (or even a group of joints), and taking it through a wide range of motion (ROM) to a point just slightly beyond where you might normally find it comfortable. This point should not be too far, where pain is felt, but to a level where there is slight discomfort. Once this point is attained, the stretch should be held for a period of time to be effective.

Dynamic stretching is a different approach to enhance flexibility. The focus on the joint involves mimicking a particular exercise movement but at a much lower level of intensity than you would when exercising. This type of stretching is used to warm up the joints, and reduce muscle tension or stiffness, prior to exercising.

We will review these approaches in more detail when we cover stretching techniques in a later chapter. For now, it is important to remember that the objective is to try and increase your ROM over time and not during any one workout - it takes time, practice and patience!

There are anatomical muscle charts on pages 36 and 37 that will help you understand the location and movement of many muscles of the body.

The following list of joints, and associated ROM, are provided as a guide to assist with you with determining your individual flexibility. Keep in mind that everyone has varying degrees of natural flexibility. I have also included photographs to illustrate each movement and to provide you with some additional assistance in identifying your ROM.

Please note that the photographs are not intended to provide the Typical ROM for each joint noted below. They are shown to provide an understanding of the "types of joint movements" only.

Joint	Type of Movement	Typical ROM
Shoulder	Flexion	90 degrees
	Extension	45 degrees
	Abduction	90 degrees
	Horizontal Extension	90 degrees
	Horizontal Flexion	90 degrees
Elbow	Flexion	150 degrees
Spine	Flexion	60 degrees
	Extension	25 degrees
	Lateral Flexion	25 degrees
Hip	Flexion	125 degrees
	Extension	15 degrees
	Abduction	45 degrees
	Hyper-extension	15 degrees
Knee	Flexion	130 degrees
Ankle	Dorsi-flexion	20 degrees
	Plantar Flexion	50 degrees
Wrist	Flexion	60 degrees
	Hyper-extension	60 degrees

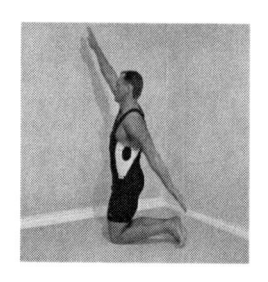

Shoulder Flexion (upper arm)
Shoulder Extension (lower arm)

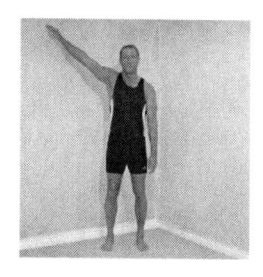

Shoulder Abduction

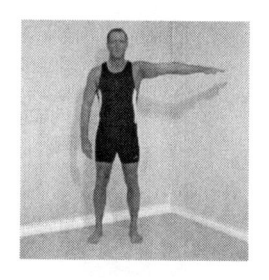

Shoulder Horizontal Extension

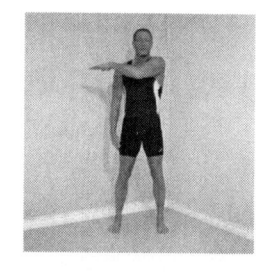

Shoulder Horizontal Flexion

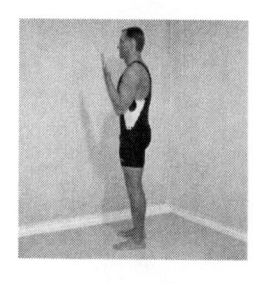

Elbow Flexion

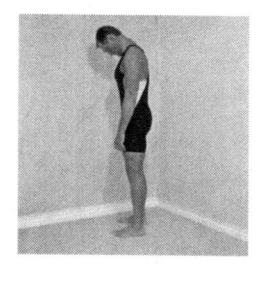

Spine Flexion

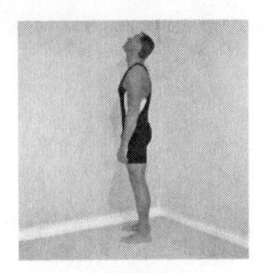

Spine Extension

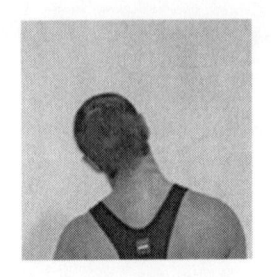

Spine Lateral Flexion

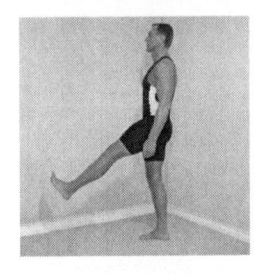

Hip Flexion

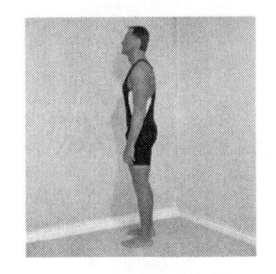

Hip Extension

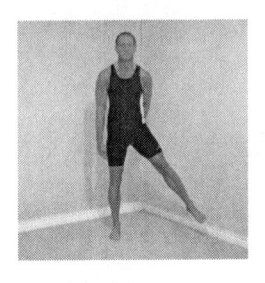

Hip Abduction

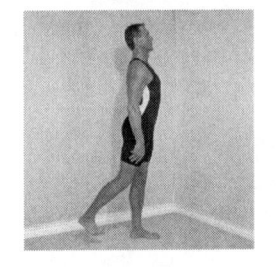

Hip Hyper Extension

REAR ANATOMICAL CHART

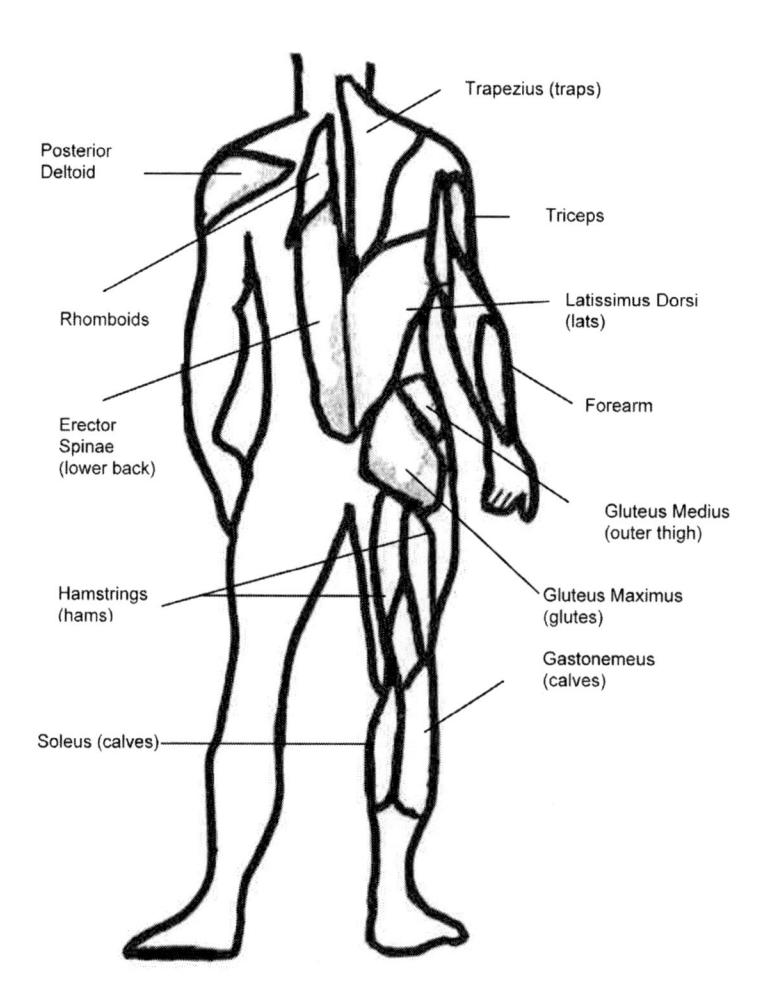

- Posterior Deltoid
- Trapezius (traps)
- Triceps
- Rhomboids
- Latissimus Dorsi (lats)
- Forearm
- Erector Spinae (lower back)
- Gluteus Medius (outer thigh)
- Hamstrings (hams)
- Gluteus Maximus (glutes)
- Gastonemeus (calves)
- Soleus (calves)

Copyright: Weight lossresources.co.uk/exercise/muscles/muscle_diagram.htm

DO YOU HAVE GOOD EATING HABITS?

Nutrition is typically not given the proper attention it deserves yet it is an important element of any physically demanding program. A well defined nutrition program can assist with muscle and cardiovascular development. It can help repair muscle tissue and speed up the recovery process when the body is challenged with extended physically demanding activity.

Before starting a fitness program you may want to seriously consider evaluating your nutritional balance. Nutritional balance is your ability to make intelligent and informed dietary choices that will help with your fitness. Even if you are already fit, it can help maintain an even healthier and energetic lifestyle. Like any car, the body requires fuel to operate. Higher octane fuels and additives typically improve the performance of a car. The body is no different in that it will perform better when supplemented with proper nutrition.

To help provide you with some basic understanding of your own nutritional balance, consider your answers to the following questions:

1. Do I have variety in what I eat?

2. Each day do I eat 3 to 5 servings of different fruits and vegetables?

3. On a daily basis, do I eat 5 to 12 servings of grain products?

4. Do I have 2 to 4 servings of milk (low fat) products daily?

5. Do I eat 2 to 3 servings of meat each day?

6. Are beans and legumes part of my diet?

7. Do I eat fish/seafood at least once a week?

8. Do I take vitamin supplements to help my diet?

9. Do I stay away from fast food outlets?

Once you have completed your own brief review, you may want to engage a qualified dietician/nutritionist. Another option might be to ask your family physician to conduct a more detailed nutritional evaluation. Additionally, I have provided some brief guidance concerning nutrition in the last chapter of this guide.

WHAT "TRAINING ZONE" SHOULD YOU USE?

I mentioned previously that it is important to understand your Resting Heart Rate, your Maximum Heart Rate and your Training Heart Rate Zone prior to exercising. You need to know the first two heart rates before you can determine your Training Heart Rate Zone. The **Resting Heart Rate** (RHR) is just what it implies: it is the number of times the heart beats per minute when the body is at complete rest.

To determine your RHR, check your pulse for 30 seconds in the morning when you first wake up and before you get out of bed. When you are counting, the first beat will count as zero. To determine the beats per minute (bpm), simply multiply your count by 2. One place where you can check your heart rate is the carotid artery. You do this by placing your index and middle finger on the side of your neck just below your jaw line (close to your throat).

A heart rate monitor can also be used to measure both resting and exercise heart rates, however, some professionals suggest a monitor may not be very accurate. As you increase your fitness level your RHR gradually decreases. However, RHR does tend to increase with age. Normally, the Resting Heart Rate for men is about 70 bpm and for women is around 75 bpm.

Research has shown that there is a relationship between exercise intensity and heart beat. The **Maximum Heart Rate** of an individual is determined by simply deducting your age from 220. For example, if you are 54 years old, your theoretical maximum heart rate, when exercising, is 166. Although it may not necessarily be the best approach, maximum heart rate can be used to help determine your level of exercise intensity (I would, however, suggest it be used as a guide only).

Professionals usually recommend a more personal approach for determining your exercise intensity based on heart rate. It involves two separate calculations that include three pieces of information: 1) your maximum heart rate; 2) your resting heart rate; and 3) the exercise intensity level you chose to work at. This information, combined with specific formulae, determines the **Training Heart Rate Zone** or the upper and lower range of heart rates that you can safely work within when exercising.

This range provides a guide to help you know how hard you should exercise for cardiovascular gain but not take you beyond a point where there are diminishing returns (due to the body being unable to provide enough energy to maintain a good workout).

Before you calculate your Training Heart Rate Zone there are other types of heart rate zones that you should understand, like your "warm up zone" and "cool down zone". Many practitioners suggest that when you are warming up, in preparation for exercise, you should try to attain a heart rate of approximately 50-60% of your maximum heart rate. Similarly, when you are cooling down after a workout you should strive for the same rate.

In terms of your "training zone", and depending on your level of fitness, many professionals suggest a range for workout intensity between 50-90% of your maximum heart rate. I have read some publications that suggest levels even as high as 95%. Given this wide variance, I recommend the following training zone guidelines:

1. **Beginners and Warm Up** - individuals with little exercise experience might begin training in the 50-60% range of maximum heart rate. This level of exercise intensity will improve cardio fitness for those beginning a fitness

program. This range is also a good guideline for warm ups for individuals at a higher level of fitness.

2. **Fitness Level** – individuals who are at a moderate level of fitness and are looking for more intensity can train in the 60-70% range of maximum heart rate level. This level of intensity typically increases caloric burn and tones muscles.

3. **Aerobic Intensity** - for individuals who are more advanced or want to perform endurance training, the 70-80% range of maximum heart rate level is ideal. Training in this zone will improve your cardiovascular and respiratory systems.

4. **Anaerobic Intensity** - for those that want to train at a very intense level they may select the 80-90% zone. This level of exercise intensity is typically reserved for the seasoned athlete who is looking to improve endurance while maximizing the burning of calories. Before training at this level, you should already be in excellent condition and perhaps even consult your family doctor.

Although the training zones noted above increase by increments of 10%, it does not mean that you could not select different ranges (50-55bpm or 55-65bpm) if they are found to be more suitable for you. Keep in mind these are general guidelines. Depending on the individual, and their health status, these ranges may also fluctuate somewhat after consulting with a family doctor.

To provide you with some direction for applying the above guidelines, let's assume we have a 54 year old that has not worked out before, has a resting heart rate of 68 and would like to improve his/her physical condition. This would mean the individual would try working out as a Beginner in the 50-60% range to start with. The following shows how to calculate his or her training zone:

The **lower value** of the range for this individual, applying the 50% exercise intensity level and a resting heart rate of 68, would be as follows:

(Max Heart Rate − Age − Resting Heart Rate) X Exercise Intensity + Resting Heart Rate

(220 bpm − 54 years old − 68 bpm) X 50% + 68

Lower Value bpm = 117 bpm

The **upper value** of the range for this individual, applying the 60% exercise intensity level, would be as follows:

(Max Heart Rate − Age − Resting Heart Rate) X Exercise Intensity + Resting Heart Rate

(220 bpm − 54 years old − 68 bpm) X 60% + 68

Upper Value bpm = 126.8 bpm

The training zone for this individual is between 117 − 127 bpm.

The lower level of the Training Heart Rate Zone tends to decrease as your level of fitness improves. This is because your heart becomes stronger and your Resting Heart Rate becomes lower. Essentially, the heart needs to work even harder for the body to maintain or improve the level of exercise intensity. The upper level of the range also decreases because the heart does not work as hard since it has become more accustomed to exercise.

To help illustrate the above points, let's follow the earlier example and assume our Beginner, after 3 months of dedicated training, has improved his/her fitness level and now has a resting heart rate of 55.

If the intensity level is left at 50-60%, the target training zone changes as shown below. Because the heart rate range is now lower, the individual does not have to work as hard as in the past to stay in the training zone and will actually get less out of their exercising unless modifications are made to intensity level. Cardiovascular gains previously realized could begin to deteriorate because the body has become used to working at this level.

Lower Value

(Max Heart Rate − Age − Resting Heart Rate) X Exercise Intensity + Resting Heart Rate

(220 bpm − 54 years of age − 55 bpm) X 50% + 55

Lower Value bpm = 110.5 bpm

Upper Value

(Max Heart Rate − Age − Resting Heart Rate) X Exercise Intensity + Resting Heart Rate

(220 bpm − 54 years of age − 55 bpm) X 60% + 55

Upper Value bpm = 121.6 bpm

The training zone has changed to 111 – 122 bpm.

To continue on with this example, changes should be made to the exercise intensity level so the "once beginner" may progress even further in terms of fitness. If the next level of exercise intensity (Fitness Level: 60-70%) is applied, you can see that the training zone moves higher. The individual in this example will continue to realize cardiovascular gain if he or she now exercises within the new training zone that has been modified due to his/her improved fitness (122-133 bpm).

Lower Value (increase intensity)

(Max Heart Rate − Age − Resting Heart Rate) X Exercise Intensity + Resting Heart Rate

(220 bpm − 54 years of age − 55 bpm) X 60% + 55

Lower Value bpm = 121.6 bpm

Upper Value (increase intensity)

(Max Heart Rate − Age − Resting Heart Rate) X Exercise Intensity + Resting Heart Rate

(220 bpm − 54 years of age − 55 bpm) X 70% + 55

Upper Value bpm = 132.7 bpm

The training zone has changed to 122 − 133 bpm.

Once again, it is important to continually review your goals, and even the fitness program you have created. Once goals or certain training levels are achieved the body requires further challenges so that it does not become too comfortable with certain exercises or programs.

FULL BODY EXERCISE FORMAT

There are numerous types of exercises and interesting programs included in this guide that will challenge you while providing variety in your workout. Aside from the vast array of exercises you can draw from to create your own program, there are many specific types of workouts that involve full body balanced programs, speed and agility, cross training and cardio challenges. All of the programs and special workouts provided follow the same general format to ensure you have a balanced full body workout. These workouts consist of the following elements, each of which will be addressed in detail:

1. Warm up
2. Cardiovascular training
3. Resistance training for the upper body, lower body and the core
4. Flexibility and cool down.

WARM UP

Eating a good breakfast is important to start the day and, likewise, properly warming up is important to start a workout. There does not have to be a set format just so long as you are warming up your joints, your muscles and your body in general. To determine if you have completed an effective warm up, you should feel the following: 1) your body feels warm; 2) your breathing is faster and; 3) your heart rate has elevated to 50-60% of your maximum heart rate.

If you prefer to perform some type of stretching at this stage of your workout, you could do so provided your joints and muscles are warmed up. I recommend staying with the dynamic stretching suggestions, provided in the upcoming Warm Up section, included in the exercise chapter. They are focused more on preparing the body for the actual movements that will be applied during your workout.

In case you are not convinced of the importance of a warm up, the following are some additional reasons for performing a warm up prior to exercising:

1. It reduces the chance of injury to muscles and joints and increases strength and speed.

2. It warms up the nervous system. This produces better strength, speed and coordination.

3. Warming up allows the body to gear up and deliver more oxygen to working muscles to assist with a better workout.

4. It will help prevent early fatigue.

5. It reduces stress on the cardiovascular system by taking the body from rest to exercise mode in a slow but moderate fashion.

A warm up should not place demands on the body. It is simply a means to prepare the body for the "work" it is about to do. There are a number of techniques that are provided within this guide to assist with a proper warm up. Many of them involve dynamic stretching and integration techniques. These approaches are designed to increase the full range of motion of a joint through active movement.

CARDIOVASCULAR TRAINING

Cardiovascular training helps to improve cardio (heart) and vascular (circulatory system) capacity. In doing so, it helps provide you with a stronger heart while reducing your resting heart rate and normalizing blood pressure. According to the American Sports Medicine Institute (ASMI), "cardiovascular fitness is a special form of muscular endurance". They further define it as "the efficiency of the heart, lungs, and vascular system in delivering oxygen to the working muscle tissues so that prolonged physical work can be maintained". It improves your ability to perform daily normal activities as well as giving you the ability to undertake more strenuous workouts. With the ability to conduct more challenging workouts, your muscular and cardiovascular development is also enhanced. Some of the other benefits of a good cardiovascular workout include the following:

1. Provides a flow of oxygen and nutrients to the body and working muscles, while improving waste removal.

2. Strengthens the heart muscle so that it can pump more blood per heart beat. This is important for overall development.

3. Increases protein substances enhancing the body's ability to use oxygen.

4. Helps improve leanness and body composition.

Due to these reasons, cardiovascular training is a key component of any physical fitness program that should not be omitted. If you are ever constrained with time to complete your entire workout, I would strongly encourage you NOT to cut back on the cardio component.

RESISTANCE (STRENGTH) TRAINING

Every movement of the body requires some kind of muscle movement. Muscles are attached to the bones in your body and you need the muscle to move your bone or joint.

Muscles are very sensitive to training in terms of growth and development. As they grow larger and stronger, they make it easier to perform movements. This is why it is especially important for athletes to have strength in their muscles for the sport they enjoy since it makes it easier for them to perform the movements they require to excel.

Many people seem to have the impression that only athletes require muscle mass or well toned bodies. Athletes do require more muscle mass but that is because of the greater demands they place on their muscles compared with people in general. The average person needs muscle mass too, but for different and equally important reasons like working around the house and yard. Generally speaking, everyone's muscles need to be challenged. Increasing muscle mass:

1. Reduces the potential for muscle and joint injury;

2. Improves strength and posture;

3. Creates a strong and toned physique;

4. Makes regular day-to-day activities easier to perform;

5. Helps prevent osteoporosis;

6. Helps keep you leaner and more physically fit because muscles utilize more calories than fat;

7. Improves strength for extended cardio exercise and further caloric burn.

FLEXIBILITY

After a workout, it is necessary to help your body recover so that it is prepared to respond to the demands placed upon it during the next workout. This is a great time to perform flexibility training, or stretching, as the muscles are warm and they are prepared to be stretched to a whole new level. This is also a good time to conduct a proper cool down. I find it challenging to talk about cooling down from a workout without including it in a discussion involving stretching. Stretching and cooling down go together to help prepare the body for the next workout and allow for even greater challenges that will encourage improvements in cardiovascular and resistance (strength) training).

Some of the key benefits of flexibility training include:

1. Assists with posture that is especially crucial in the development of young adolescents;

2. Lengthens the muscles and maintains durability;

3. Improves performance associated with everyday activities, sports and exercise;

4. Reduces the risk of injury;

5. Reduces stress while exercising muscles, and releasing tension;

6. Promotes a relaxed mood that helps the body recover while assisting with improved sleep patterns.

Stretching should always be performed at the end of a session as a cool down to increase flexibility and to enhance cardio and resistance training. **Please also note that stretching should be performed to a level of discomfort only.** Going beyond that may increase the risk of injury so please exercise caution. The duration, number and type of individual stretches you perform are typically consistent with the intensity of your workout and those muscles that you work. A simple rule of thumb is to stretch those muscles that were impacted by your workout. The stretches provided later in this guide identify the major muscles being stretched by each technique to provide you some assistance. Although there are differing opinions on this topic, a good rule of thumb is to hold each stretch for 25-30 seconds.

COOL DOWN

Lactic acid tends to build up in the muscles and blood from continuous exertion. It causes slower body and muscle movement as a result. If you do nothing after a workout, your body does not receive the proper amounts of oxygen required to replenish muscle stores of energy and remove lactic acid and other waste. Lactic acid needs to be removed to avoid muscle cramping and promote muscle recovery so they are prepared to provide energy when needed next time. If not done properly, muscles may show signs of fatigue or just simply not respond adequately when needed. A good way to help your body return to a "post workout" state and help remove lactic acid is to include a "cool down" drill in the stretching component of your workout.

It is important to breathe properly while you are working out and it is equally important to apply proper breathing techniques when cooling down. Diaphragmatic breathing is an effective way of breathing while exercising and it is equally effective for a cool down or relaxation. It involves using your diaphragm to breathe instead of your chest. You will know if you are breathing this way when your stomach rises instead of your chest expanding. This breathing technique will increase the efficiency of your lungs and help improve your recovery.

While you are performing stretching, you should practice breath control ("Pranayama – the art of Yoga breathing" as stated by ABC of Yoga. com). When you start with an "open form" type of stretch, like a Full Body stretch, inhale and continue with slow and easy breathing that involves breathing in and out to a count of three. When you perform a "closed form" type of stretch, like the Rollerball, start with an exhale and continue with slow and easy breathing again to a three count of three in and out. Once you are comfortable with this pace, increase your inhale and exhale count to five. Regardless of the count, the key is "slow and easy breathing". Even though a good stretching session can help relax the body, and gradually bring the heart rate down to normal levels, controlled breathing helps.

Another approach you may find effective is to perform a cool down in the dark. This can help relax you, and in some class settings, I have experienced some students fall asleep during the process.

When you are cooling down, you should strive for a heart rate that is 50-60% of your maximum heart rate. This is essentially the same rate you were striving for during your warm up.

TRAINING PROGRAM METHODOLOGY

This guide has been designed to incorporate various types of methodologies and approaches towards training in an effort to continually challenge the body and enhance fitness level. The wide variety is also intended to maintain interest.

As a participant, I encourage you to periodically (perhaps every two or three weeks) do something very different and personally challenging in terms of physical fitness, like running a longer route, taking a day long bike trip or doing a long and challenging hike. It is simply a matter of what suits you, your surroundings and your own level of personal fitness at the time. You might also consider taking a day off **each week** from the program and just do some other leisure activity, like cycling, hiking, skiing, swimming, squash, soccer or skating. This is a form of "active rest" that is beneficial for your recovery, and any fresh air activity you can take in has its own benefits!

The following are brief explanations of the fitness methodologies utilized in this guide to help provide some understanding of what is included in the exercises and programs that will follow.

ENHANCED REPETITIONS & SETS

In order to continue to challenge the body in terms of resistance and cardiovascular training, we "overload" it by increasing the level of intensity over time. This is a fairly traditional approach that is done through increasing repetitions (reps), sets and the duration of particular exercises or drills as the body becomes used to higher levels of work.

A repetition is a certain movement or range of motion (ROM) that is undertaken for a particular drill or exercise. For example, when performing a push up, the up motion followed by the down motion completes the full repetition and ROM for this exercise.

A set is a number of consecutive reps completed for a particular exercise, for example 5 consecutive push ups is 1 set of 5. Program content will typically build up additional sets while increasing reps for each set. In between each of the sets there will be a short break or active rest. The length of the break normally depends on the intensity level and the number of sets and reps undertaken.

SUPERSETS

This is another approach that helps challenge the body and "overload" it. It can be accomplished in a number of different ways. Generally, the objective is to deny the body complete rest, and provide anaerobic challenge, while placing additional load on it. Initially the approach could be done aggressively for short periods.

This method can involve a number of different approaches or exercise mix. It can combine multiple upper body resistance exercises without rest between reps and sets. Another approach combines numerous upper body and lower body exercises together without rest. An even greater challenge could combine upper and lower body exercises with abs, and even plyometrics or cardio, without rest between the different types of exercise. The latter would be the most demanding and in doing so you would probably reduce the number of reps/sets performed. These are just a few approaches to give you an idea of how the method can be applied. There are endless combinations of exercises and exercise types which can be created.

EXERCISE MIXING

This is an approach that involves changing the order of specific exercises normally completed within a workout. You might be performing the cardio component of a workout but change the order, duration and intensity of the cardio exercises themselves. Another mixing technique involves mixing cardio and strength techniques within the same workout, for example a spot run followed with push ups and then sit ups or vice versa. The principle being applied involves surprising the body so it has to work harder to do something new that it is not used to.

EXERCISE & DRILL BUILDING (STACKING)

This is an effective challenge for the body that enhances coordination, endurance, muscle development and toning. Essentially it involves adding an exercise or drill to another exercise or drill previously used on its own, and executing them together. As an example, combine a Standard Squat or Lunge with Shoulder Circles (to be covered later). Another more intense example would involve a Jumping Jack and a Standard Squat executed continuously one after the other. This is an effective approach to enhance fat burning and help improve coordination.

INTERVAL TRAINING

Interval training is a high impact approach to physical fitness that involves numerous exercises, focused on different parts of the body, conducted at high intensity for a short period. Once a certain number of exercises are completed, they are followed immediately by low intensity exercise to provide for active rest and allow for sufficient recovery. Some professionals may call it Turbulence Training or Extreme Turbulence Training. Recovery time is typically dependant on your fitness level but is long enough so that you can perform the next set of high intensity drills at a maximum level. The number of sets is also dependant on your level of fitness.

Interval training is an effective way to promote anaerobic conditioning, to boost metabolism and enhance fat burning. It is not intended to improve endurance but to enhance performance so that higher intensity can be maintained for a longer period, for example sprinting for 15 seconds versus 10 seconds at the same level of intensity. Some examples of high intensity activities include soccer, football or hockey, where short spurts of energy are required.

When you use interval training, follow the general guideline below in terms of the duration of each exercise:

Beginner – 10-15 seconds
Intermediate – 30-45 seconds
Advanced – 60 seconds plus

To provide you with a greater appreciation for this type of training, the following is an example of one segment for a beginner. It involves a "full body" workout approach (warm up and cool down are not shown but are always expected) Note that each exercise would be executed for 10-15 seconds (as noted above) before moving to the next one;

1. Squats – works the legs after a warm up
2. Push ups - works the shoulders/arms while resting the legs
3. Spot run or sprint – cardio and leg work while resting the upper body
4. Ab crunches – works the abdominals while resting the lower body
5. Jog for 10-15 seconds (dependant on fitness level and/or the challenge you want for your workout) – active rest
6. First Interval Set complete

Upon completion of the first set, different exercises would be utilized for the second set but the muscle group focus, for example your legs, would be the same. Instead of a squat, a lunge might be performed. For the upper body, a different type of push up could be done, and so on.

The amount of time you spend on each, and the number of sets and exercises performed, is consistent with your level of fitness and how much you want to push yourself. This is a great cardio workout and fat burner. A sample program is included later in this guide.

CIRCUIT TRAINING

Circuit Training is one of the "top workout trends" that combines strength training with cardiovascular drills. It is another form of high impact training that involves a series of exercises using numerous parts of the body in succession. Although very similar to Interval Training, the approach is slightly different. The key difference is that a series of exercises are focused on one muscle or area of the body, followed by a type of cardio drill, before moving to the next series that has a different focus.

Similar to Interval Training, these types of workouts are typically shorter in duration, due to their high impact. Active rest is provided by moving to different muscle groups for each exercise performed without stopping in between. Individual exercises can be executed for a specific duration of time, or perhaps a selected number of reps. In either situation, you select something that challenges you and overloads your muscles.

If you are not familiar with this type of training, it may be somewhat confusing (a sample program is also provided later on). To illustrate, the following is an example of one segment that would be part of a longer Circuit Drill. This particular segment would apply to an intermediate full body workout (30-45 seconds in duration or 15-20 reps for each exercise shown);

1. Standard push ups
2. Arm Pulls
3. Tricep push ups
4. Scooping push ups
5. Dips
6. Spot jog (10 seconds) and jump – repeat for 1 minute
7. First Circuit Set complete – move to next set

The next set, following the above example, might focus on your legs, and a final set might focus on your abs and waist. The number of sets, exercises and duration would be dependant on your level of fitness. This method is another good way to burn fat.

"SHOCK" TREATMENT

The theory behind "shock treatment" is to stimulate working muscles and create a new positive overload or challenge to the muscle. Essentially, you want to catch your body off guard by giving it a "wake up" call.

With any type of training, your body eventually gets used to the movements being performed. When this happens, your body is not challenged and does not work as hard. Your level of fitness can actually diminish over time if you do not continually give it new challenges and/or variety in what you do in terms of fitness.

Basically, "shock treatment" involves continually changing exercises, drills, order, frequency, application, and so forth, so that the body does not get used to what it is doing. This constant change is also good because it keeps us from getting bored!

FOCUSED WORKOUT SESSIONS

Upon reaching a higher level of fitness you might consider expanding the number of workouts per week. These additional workouts may include enhanced focus and intensity on particular areas of development, like cardio training one day or resistance training another. For example, if you chose to focus on cardio one day, you could combine it with another training method such as Interval Training. Since a cardio workout usually involves the legs, and especially the larger muscles like the quads and glutes, you could intensify the focus of the workout, by also performing larger muscle exercises, like squats and/or lunges.

If you chose upper body resistance training for your workout, you might decide to work your arms and pecs only and even apply "Enhanced Reps" or "Exercise Building (Stacking)" to enhance the session. This approach is a positive way of testing the body, and the progress you have reached, while adding variety.

EXERCISE PREPARATION

The first thing to remember once you have decided to take on any fitness program is that it will require higher levels of energy. To exert energy, you require fuel for your body, no different than gasoline for a car as mentioned previously. There are some key steps you should take to help you prepare so you can get the most out of your exercise program.

Start by ensuring your body remains adequately hydrated at all times with water. Second, follow a proper nutritionally balanced diet. In the previous chapter, you considered questions designed to create awareness about your eating habits. A proper diet does not necessarily mean limiting your food intake or starving yourself. It means making healthy choices and consuming reasonable portions relative to your stage of life. If you are still growing or involved with high energy activities, your food intake will be higher. However, healthy eating is a habit so you will still want to be conscious of the choices you make that may come back to haunt you in your later years when your metabolism declines.

A car cannot run at high speed all the time without periodic maintenance (rest). Your body is no different. It is important that you provide your body adequate rest, otherwise, it will be difficult to maintain a vigorous workout while keeping up with other activities, like work and/or school.

HYDRATION

Approximately 60% of our body weight consists of water and for this reason alone it becomes an essential ingredient for day to day living. Water is also a good body coolant, like anti-freeze in a car, and a good lubricant for the body.

Numerous periodicals suggest, on average, that a person should drink approximately 8-12 cups (250 ml per cup) of water a day to help replace the approximate 10 cups of water lost through daily routine activities. Although not specifically covered in this book, regular water consumption assists with flushing your system routinely and also helps remove toxins from the body. The first sign of dehydration is when you become thirsty. Typically, this will occur even before your mouth starts to feel dry. To help avoid dehydration, it is good to drink water before any thirst begins to set in. Since even more water is lost during exercise, it is necessary to have a regular intake of water during a workout session, like small drinks between exercises.

The following is a suggested guideline for water intake over the course of a normal day, a day that doesn't even include exercise:

1. 500 ml (2 cups or 1 bottle) before breakfast or before you eat anything to help get your system functioning first thing in the morning
2. 500 ml with your mid-morning snack or meal
3. 500 ml with your lunch
4. 500 ml with your mid-afternoon snack or meal
5. 500 ml with your dinner

NUTRITION

Simply put, if you do not ingest the proper nutrients (carbohydrates, protein, fat, vitamins, minerals and water) through a balanced diet, you will not have the energy to sustain a demanding workout. One of the most important aspects about nutrition involves clean eating concepts. The purpose of this section is to create general awareness about nutrition since it is a key element in creating energy to help you carry out an effective workout.

Although everyone is different, a typical balanced diet consists of a good mix of carbohydrates (carbs), protein and fat. Carbs are divided into two types, simple and complex. Simple carbs consist of foods like marmalade, juices, and fruits to name a few. Complex carbs consist of foods like rice, vegetables, and beans. The best sources of carbs are those that are natural, like dairy, fruits and vegetables, since they also contain other essential fibers, minerals and vitamins. For additional assistance with developing personal dietary requirements you could search the Internet for ideas.

The average person needs about 1.0 gram of protein per day, for every kilogram of body weight, if they want to sustain their present weight. If you are a more active individual, typically you would require additional protein simply because you are burning up more energy. Like carbs, there are two types of protein sources. One is called a complete protein and the other an incomplete protein. Complete proteins come from animal protein and include fish, poultry, pork and beef. Incomplete proteins are those that do not contain essential amino acids, for example seeds, grains and nuts.

A small amount of fat is important in most diets because it provides fatty acids that are required for cell membranes and certain bodily functions. These functions include the transportation of fat soluble vitamins, like vitamins A, D, and E.

Since your body is not capable of making vitamins you need to have them provided through your diet. Vitamins are necessary for the metabolism of fats and carbs even though they do not provide any level or source of energy. Some minerals and vitamins interact with one another. There are many opinions on the use of vitamins and I suggest you consult your doctor prior to using them.

Minerals are a simple and important nutrient because they can assist the body with many different functions including body fluid balance, heart rate, bone health, muscle relaxation and transportation of oxygen through the body. Some examples of minerals include potassium, sodium, calcium, phosphorus and iron. Most minerals can be provided through a balanced diet but there are times when there may be deficiencies due to medical issues. When this is the case, it is important to consult a physician to address the problem.

REST

Ensuring you get adequate daily rest is essential for your personal health and to help you have a successful fitness program. If you do not get the proper rest to revitalize your mind and body, you will not have adequate energy. You will feel tired even before you begin your workout and you will not be in the mood (mind or body) to physically challenge yourself.

Rest times for individuals may vary based on their own specific needs. Typically, I think adolescents should get at least 9-10 hours of sleep daily and adults around 7-8 hours, especially while participating in sporting activities and other fitness programs. Some research suggests that a minimum of 9 hours sleep per day for adults is necessary if they exercise on a frequent basis. You will need to decide what works best for you.

I encourage you to keep the above three elements, hydration, nutrition and rest, in mind to help build and maintain your energy level. This is essential to sustain maximum effort when you exercise.

Although this all sounds fairly straightforward, if you chose to ignore the suggestions made about hydration, nutrition and rest, they can have an adverse affect on your progress towards achieving your goals. It could even become your recipe for failure if you end up withdrawing from your fitness program due to little or no progress, fatigue, loss of interest, or all of the above.

SET YOUR GOALS

When you have completed your self assessment, and gained a further understanding of yourself, it is time to establish your goals and make a formal commitment to your program. Consistent with setting business or personal goals or objectives, it is also necessary to do the same in terms of fitness.

It doesn't matter what type of goals you establish. They should always be specific in terms of your focus and what you want to accomplish. You also need to be able to measure progress against your goals so that you know if gains are being made, like measuring your waistline on a monthly basis.

The effort you put forth and the activities you perform need to address your area of focus and the goals you are trying to accomplish. In other words, there needs to be a direct correlation between effort-activities and focus-goals. Goals should be realistic, achievable and always challenging. Unrealistic goals can frustrate and even eliminate the personal drive to achieve results and be successful. Last but not least, efforts or activities undertaken to achieve results should always be based on a set timeframe. This will help motivate you to exert the energy required to reach the milestone or goal you set for yourself. An example of this might include you finishing a marathon in less than four hours.

The following are some sample goals that you might have after completing your health and fitness review:

1. Improve flexibility in the shoulders and hips.

2. Reduce Resting Heart Rate.

3. Decrease waist and increase chest measurements.

4. Run a longer distance in a shorter time.

5. Decrease recovery time (time to return to normal heart rate).

The fitness program that you create should align with the goals that you set for yourself. If one of your goals is to increase the number of proper form push ups you can complete then some of the exercises within your program need to include some upper body exercises, for example dips, push ups.

Your goals should always be based on your individual needs and not what others expect or feel you need to do. In an article published in the American College of Sports Medicine (ACSM) Health & Fitness Journal, the authors examined exercise motivation by looking at self-determination theory. They found that individuals are more successful in exercise programs when motivation is internal (enjoyment, personal satisfaction), rather than external (weight management, body dissatisfaction). It may be worthwhile to consider this finding when developing your personal goals.

Since noticeable gains towards improved levels of fitness are typically realized about every 2-4 weeks, it is necessary to review your goals periodically and potentially modify them so you are continually challenged. As goals are modified, you may also need to modify your program to match your goals (normally every 6-12 weeks) depending on your progress and your area of focus (upper or lower body strength, cardiovascular capacity, abs, flexibility).

TRACK YOUR PROGRESS

Now that you have set your goals, you need to track your progress. This is a crucial aspect of your program as it will help you determine if your program requires adjustment. It is also good to have a report card on yourself that you can periodically review. Tracking your progress will help you understand if your progress is falling short or where gains are being made. It will highlight areas that are working well and those that are not and, as a result, help you determine what modifications you may need to make to your program.

While you need to track your progress, and make changes as required, it is also important to be patient with your program. You do not want to be making numerous changes to it without first giving it a chance to work. However, as you achieve higher levels of fitness, you may want to consider changes on a more frequent basis to provide yourself with greater anaerobic challenges.

If you are not realizing the gains you would like to see after staying with your program for a reasonable time, you may want to ask yourself:

1. Am I working hard enough and giving the effort required (check to see if your Training Heart Rate zone is too low)?

2. Do I need to increase the reps, time or effort I apply to a specific exercise?

3. Am I getting enough rest?

4. Do I have enough exercises included in my workout or am I working out long enough?

5. Do I have the right mix of exercises?

6. Am I staying with my program?

7. Do I follow proper form for each exercise?

8. Do I have a typical daily training time and overall schedule?

9. Do I have healthy eating habits and am I consuming the right food?

If you decide that modifications are required to your program, you should revisit your goals to ensure they are in alignment with any changes you have made. Thereafter, you can re-establish your starting point and continue to monitor your progress against your new goals.

To help you accurately track your progress I have designed a **Progress Tracking Sheet**. Blank copies of this form are provided at the end of this guide for your use (you may want to make copies of the blank form or "enlarge them" before marking them up). The forms allow enough space for you to record and track your progress over a 12 week period. This gives you the opportunity to plot your progress for a reasonable period of time while showing you the impact of any program changes or modifications you made (remember, you should be reviewing your program and goals about every 6 weeks).

On the following page is a sample **Progress Tracking Sheet** which is intended to give you some guidance in terms of how to fill it out. It allows you to list the exercises that are part of your program and track the reps and sets you perform on a weekly basis (always striving to do better, daily and/or weekly). As a point of clarification, the notation "1X10", as shown for Squats, means that you perform 1 set of 10 reps for that particular exercise. In terms of clarity, the rest of the form is fairly straightforward.

SAMPLE - Personal Program Progress Track Sheet

Date: June 1, 20___

Warm Up (3 - 5 min.) – Options: Spot run or jog or cycle; integrators, neck rotations, leg/shoulder circles

Cardio – Options: Run, cycle, swim, stair climb, treadmill or a combination (always change it up)

Exercise/Drill	June REPS x SETS	June	June	June	July	July	July	July	August	August	August	August
Squat	1x10	1x11	1x12	1x13	1x14	1x15	1x16	1x17	1x18	1x19	1x20	1x21
Front Lunge	1x6	1x7	1x8	1x9	1x10	1x11	1x12	1x13	1x14	1x15	1x16	1x17
Side Lunge	1x8	1x8	1x8	1x8	2x8	2x8	2x8	2x8	3x8	3x8	3x8	3x8
Jumping Jacks												
Front Kick												
Side Kick												
Standard Push up												
Perfect Push up												
Dip												
Sit up												
Leg Raise												
Side Bend												
Side Crunch												
Glute Stretch	15 sec	15 sec	15 sec	15 sec	20 sec	20 sec	20 sec	20 sec	25 sec	25 sec	25 sec	25 sec
Hamstring Stretch	1x15	1x15	1x15	1x15	2x15	2x15	2x15	2x15	2x20	2x20	2x20	2x20
Calve Stretch												
Bicep Stretch												
Tricep Stretch												

WHEN SHOULD YOU WORK OUT?

There are numerous things to consider when deciding on the best time to work out. The first consideration is to determine what works best for your own schedule. I find that having a workout first thing in the morning is ideal because the busy day has not started and there are fewer obstacles and distractions. The difficulty for some people is that getting up earlier than usual can be a challenge at first. However, once you get used to it, you are rewarded with a fresh start for the day that will actually energize you (it may, however, take 3-4 weeks to get used to a new early morning schedule). Although ideal, in my opinion, I know this may not always be practical or even possible for some people.

It may actually take a couple of weeks of trying different times to narrow down what schedule works best for you. Once you determine the optimum time of day for your workout, I highly recommend you adhere to it. This may sound trivial but it is a key element of sustaining a successful program. It is all too easy to say "I'm too busy today but I'll make it up tomorrow". Typically, tomorrow does not come. Sometimes it may be necessary to change your workout time or schedule because some days it just may not be possible to do your workout as planned. However, even if you only complete part of your workout, it is more beneficial in terms of maintaining your overall program than not doing anything at all. Obviously this is not optimal. However, it could help to keep you on track, especially in the early stages, until you establish a regular routine (this usually takes about three weeks).

There are a number of factors you should consider when you are trying to determine the best time and days to exercise:

1. **Rest** – the body needs to re-charge. When you are building muscle, cells are destroyed. They require nutrition and rest to replenish so they can get even stronger and leaner. Depending on the muscle and type of workout you have, you may need anywhere from 24-48 hours of rest (perhaps even more) for the muscle worked. Just to clarify, that does not mean you should not work out two days in a row. It just means working different muscles or groups.

2. **Muscle groups** – you may want to focus on a particular muscle or group of muscles one day (upper body or even chest and arms), versus another muscle or muscle group the next day (lower body – legs or abs).

3. **Strength versus cardio** – even though I recommend you perform a full body workout each time you exercise, your own preference may be to focus on resistance (strength) training one day and cardio capacity another if that is the type of program you chose.

4. **Type of workout and knowing your body** – another approach may involve a full body workout that includes resistance and cardio exercises individually or even combined. Some people find that cardio is easier to do in the morning or prefer it as a good wakeup. Others may feel stronger at lunch and complete resistance training then. In any case, I recommend you go with what works best for you and allows you to perform at your best.

5. **Warm Up and Cool Down** - ensure that your workouts allow for time to conduct a proper warm up and a cool down that includes some amount of stretching at the end of your workout.

6. **Area of focus** – you may have a preference to build muscle, increase leanness or perhaps even focus on your abs. This could impact the number of times per week that you work out. Additional workouts per week can help you increase leanness. On the other hand, fewer workouts, focused on a particular muscle or group of muscles, can help to increase muscle mass.

7. **Time of day** – some professionals suggest that resistance training performed first thing in the morning provides a greater opportunity for continued caloric burn through the remainder of the day. On the other hand, some individuals prefer to start the day with a steady cardio type of workout, like swimming or aerobics, as this provides them with a prolonged higher metabolism.

Generally, I suggest you try to avoid evening workouts since exercise increases metabolism. Depending on the intensity of your workout, it may take time to "cool down" and relax so you can get a good night sleep and be ready for the next day. Also be mindful that the time of day you chose to exercise needs to be balanced with the needs of your body and when it performs best.

HOW OFTEN SHOULD YOU WORKOUT?

How often you work out really depends on your individual situation but there are some general guidelines you can apply. Typically, if you exercise only once a week, you will not realize much improvement in terms of physical fitness, if anything at all. If you work out twice a week, it can help you maintain some degree of your current fitness level, and if you have never worked out previously, it can provide some minor initial gains. If you exercise a minimum of three to five times per week this typically provides continuous gain. The American College of Sports Medicine recommends that "individuals should workout three to five times per week". Working out six or seven times a week, depending on the individual, may actually hinder results while for others it might enhance progress.

The number of times you exercise each week can also be dependant on the type of program you are following. Consistent with the theme of "constant change", as a workout methodology, I suggest you shift around the days you exercise and the number of times you exercise about every 4-6 weeks. You might consider this once you reach a level of reasonable fitness. This is another way to continually challenge your body. You can also include fresh air activities, like hiking, in your program for those non-workout or active rest days.

The following pages provide some suggestions for workout schedules, and ideas for mixing up your program, based on differing levels of fitness and personal objectives. Note that a warm up, and cool down that includes stretching, should always be included in any workout even if not specifically mentioned in the following examples.

IMPROVE GENERAL FITNESS

Beginner:

Monday-Wednesday-Friday or Tuesday-Thursday-Saturday

- Full Body workout during the day with an activity over the weekend.
- Complete a 1-2 hour weekend activity like cycling, walking or hiking to include fresh air.

Intermediate:

Four Full Body workouts per week (alternate days)

- On one of the weekend days, complete a challenging 1-4 hour activity to add variety and provide cross training (cycling, running, swimming or an aerobics class).
- Try to include some fresh air in your activity.

Advanced:

Monday-Wednesday-Friday - Upper Body workout that includes the abs and;

Tuesday-Thursday-Saturday – Lower Body workout that includes the obliques and 30-45 minutes of Cardio.

- Rest on Sunday.
- If you want to be more aggressive, go without rest and complete a challenging activity on Sunday.
- An activity could involve something outside of the norm (long run; long swim; bike trip)
- The idea is to challenge the body by "shocking" it (something it is not used to). An even more aggressive activity, like running a half marathon, might be done monthly. This is really dependant on personal circumstances, fitness level and personal goals.

IMPROVE CARDIOVASCULAR CAPACITY

Beginner:

Monday-Wednesday-Friday or Tuesday-Thursday-Saturday

- Focus on Cardio training, including the abs and the obliques, every other day as shown above.
- 1-2 times per week complement the Cardio training with upper/lower body strength exercises.
- Complete a 1-2 hour activity over the weekend like cycling, walking or hiking that includes fresh air.

Intermediate:

Four workouts per week (alternate days)

- Focus on Cardio training, and include the abs and the obliques, on the days noted.
- One or two Upper/Lower Body Resistance workouts between Cardio days.
- On one of the weekend days, take in a different exercise activity from the norm like an aerobics class, long bike ride, skiing.
- Rest on Sunday.

Advanced:

Monday/Tuesday & Thursday/Friday – Lower Body workout that includes abs/obliques & 30-45 minutes of Cardio and;

Wednesday/Saturday - Full Body workout that includes the obliques and is followed by 15-20 minutes of Cardio.

- Cardio format should be different each week day.
- Complete a 2-4 hour Cardio activity Saturday for variety instead of the Cardio noted above.
- A more aggressive activity, like running a half marathon, might be done monthly.
- Active rest on Sunday like a long walk.

IMPROVE STRENGTH AND MUSCLE TONE

Beginner:

Monday-Wednesday-Friday or Tuesday-Thursday-Saturday

- Focus on Full Body Resistance training.
- 1-2 times per week complement the Full Body training with Cardio.
- Complete a 1-2 hour activity over the weekend like cycling, walking or hiking that includes fresh air.

Intermediate:

Four workouts per week (alternate days)

- Focus on Full Body Resistance training every other day.
- One or two Cardio workouts between Full Body Resistance workouts.
- On one of the weekend days, take in a different activity from the norm like an aerobics class, long run or bike ride.
- Rest on Sunday.

Advanced:

Monday/Tuesday & Thursday/Friday – Full Body Resistance workout that includes the abs/obliques and;

Wednesday/Saturday – 30-45 minute Cardio workout plus a Lower Resistance workout that includes the abs/obliques.

- A more aggressive program could include a Full Body workout on Sunday that is shorter in duration.
- Active rest on Sunday like a long walk, hike, golf.

HOW LONG SHOULD YOUR WORKOUT BE?

The amount of time you should devote to your workout is a function of several things including fitness level, your type of workout and your area of focus. Although it is preferable to stick to a schedule, my philosophy is that any time you spend doing a workout is better than doing nothing at all.

Depending on your fitness level, you may require one to three weeks to "ramp up" to the optimum time that is actually necessary for your daily workout routine to be beneficial in terms of cardiovascular gain. The number of exercises, and corresponding sets/reps, you include for an effective workout will determine the amount of time it will take. The intensity of your workout will also influence its duration. Some programs, like interval training or circuit training, can be shorter but quite intense. However, a more intense workout will require a longer cool down that incorporates more stretching. All of these factors impact the actual length of time you need to have a thorough and beneficial workout.

Generally speaking, if you have not been active in past, you should start off with 25-35 minutes of exercise 1–3 times a week. As your comfort and fitness level improves, your duration of exercise can increase. If you are a more active individual, the length of time you workout may be anywhere from 45-90 minutes. Typically, the duration of your workout increases with fitness level because your body becomes more accustomed to exercise and you will need to do more to keep it challenged.

In order to improve your cardiovascular development, you should strive for a workout that is 30-60 minutes long with a continuously elevated heart rate. Obviously, you will need to pace yourself when you first start out.

To work towards your ideal suggested workout time, I would add approximately 1-2 minutes each week to each of your workouts until you reach the level you feel will help you reach your goals.

In terms of a general guideline for the beginner, intermediate or advanced individual, the following are suggested durations for the various components of a full body workout.

Activity	**Beginner**	**Intermediate**	**Advanced**
Warm up	3-5 minutes	3-7 minutes	5-10 minutes
Cardio	10-20 minutes	20-40 minutes	40-60 minutes
Resistance (# of exercises)	5-10	10-15	15-20
Cool down	5-10 minutes	15-20 minutes	20-30 minutes

The duration of your workout may also depend on your goals and how aggressive they are. You should also factor in the appropriate amount of rest so that you do not deplete yourself or run the risk of injury.

PROPER FORM IS CRUCIAL

If you find that you perform the suggested number of repetitions of a particular exercise before you get tired, and your gain is minimal, there are several factors that could be the cause. One of these is poor form.

Typically, if you pay attention to the details associated with proper form, it will pay you dividends. It is easier to move quickly through a workout and perform all the exercises you have selected, without proper form. Furthermore, you may not feel anything in terms of muscle fatigue. As a result, you may conclude that your workout is not challenging enough or even enjoyable. However, if you take the time to perform your exercises correctly, with proper form, you will notice amazing differences over the longer term. You'll feel better about your workout and you will also be happy with your physical transformation.

When proper form is introduced, the body is challenged to a greater extent and the number of reps drops considerably before the body builds the strength to do more. The body also responds faster to proper form in terms of muscular and cardiovascular development because the muscles are being challenged.

It is easy to develop bad habits that can lead to inferior or minimal improvements to fitness. Since this is a "how to" book, my focus is to emphasize proper form for all exercises. I have included pictures of each exercise, along with detailed descriptions, that I encourage you to follow.

There are a number of topical areas that relate to form and they include things like how fast you should perform an exercise; how many reps or sets you should complete; and how you should breathe while you exercise. All of these different aspects complement one another and they will impact your level of development and progress.

HOW FAST SHOULD YOU EXECUTE AN EXERCISE?

When you conduct resistance training it is important to follow proper methods to get the best out of your workout. Working the muscle at a slower pace can help provide greater challenge for the muscles and enhance development. However, there are specific instances when you may want to increase the pace of your exercises or drills to help improve reflexes, speed and even toning.

Ideally, reps should be performed to a count of six: two counts for the concentric contraction (or "up" phase – muscle shortens) and four counts for the eccentric movement (or "down" phase – muscle lengthens) of the exercise. Maintaining this pace will allow optimal development of the muscle fibres. Muscles are stronger on the eccentric contraction (or down phase) simply because the muscle lengthens and has to work harder. You may want to experiment with different "counts" yourself to see what gives you the greater muscle "burn" when performing various exercises.

HOW MANY REPS SHOULD YOU PERFORM?

It is difficult to have a discussion involving reps without including sets. In my opinion, the number of reps you complete in your workout must be based on the assumption that you will apply the proper form to each and every exercise being executed. As you develop and improve your form over time, your number of repetitions will also increase. Reps will also be addressed in the next topic involving "sets".

As with any type of exercise, especially resistance (strength) training, the objective is to apply enough work (load) on the muscle(s) of focus so that they are forced to work harder than normal and reach a level of failure. Failure is the point where you cannot complete any more reps with proper form. The number of reps or sets you perform of a particular exercise, like a pushup, places additional load on the muscles you are working (pecs and triceps). When muscles are pushed to work harder they end up forming little rips in the muscle fibre that the body repairs. As the body repairs these fibres the muscles become larger and/or more toned.

The actual number of reps you perform will vary as you improve your level of fitness, change the type of exercise(s) you perform or make modifications to your program. You are the best judge of the number of reps you can complete, especially when you factor in how much you intend to push yourself. Typically, the number or reps you perform, or strive for, should be in the 8-25 range (remember that reps are higher because only body weight is being applied). I recommend you complete the maximum number of reps you need to in order to attain your fitness goals. In other words, make sure the number of reps fits with your program in terms of the results you want and what works best for you.

As a guideline, to increase muscle mass you would perform fewer reps, at a slower rate, and increase the number of sets. If you want to increase your muscle tone you would complete more reps, the speed between reps and fewer sets.

In closing, it is important to distinguish the number of reps that are applied to "weight training" versus what I recommend in this guide. Since weight training involves utilizing considerably more weight than the body is typically used to, fewer reps and sets are normally performed. When you are using "body weight" type exercises for the resistance applied to your muscles, the number of reps and sets increases to apply greater load. For this reason, you may notice different suggestions for exercise reps and sets in this guide than what you may be accustomed to seeing in other documentation that is more focused on weight training.

HOW MANY SETS SHOULD YOU COMPLETE?

You could increase the number of sets performed in order to add load to the muscles so they are brought to a level of failure. This is what you want for muscle development. Increasing your sets can also help you improve your technique.

As you get older, you may need to execute more sets and fewer reps to maintain muscle mass. If you are younger, you may need to execute more reps and fewer sets, depending on your focus. You can experiment with the number of reps and sets to see what works well for you once you are comfortable with the exercises in this book. Over time, as you get to know your body, its capabilities, and how far you can push it, you will come to know what works best for you.

Once you have reached the maximum level of reps suggested in the previous section (this is different for everyone in terms of the exercises chosen, and your specific program or goals), you will want to continue to challenge your muscles by adding sets to your workout. Instead of executing one exercise 10 reps, you could perform the same exercise two or three times for 10 reps each time (with defined rest in between). This will help bring your muscle(s) to a point of failure as discussed earlier.

In terms of some simple guidelines regarding sets, I recommend the following;

1. 2 sets of higher reps (12-20) to improve endurance and toning

2. 3-5 sets of lower reps (8-12) to help build strength, power and greater muscle mass

3. 5 sets of lower reps to work on form and technical details

4. A total of 15-30 sets of all the exercises in your workout (dependant on your level of fitness and the program you have chosen)

HOW SHOULD YOU BREATHE WHEN YOU EXERCISE?

A component of proper form involves breathing. It is important to breathe consistently while you exercise. When you are exerting yourself, or applying effort in performing an exercise, you should breathe out. You certainly should not hold your breath because this can increase your blood pressure. It can also increase the pressure in your chest and reduce the flow of oxygen to the brain leading to possible faintness and even passing out. The main thing to remember is to breathe consistently while you are working out so that you maintain a continual flow of oxygen to your body.

The American College of Sports Medicine states "the correct way to breathe during activity is to exhale during the most difficult portion of the exercise and inhale during the easier portion".

HINTS FOR A SUCCESSFUL PROGRAM

Unfortunately, most people give up on exercising even before it has had a chance to really work for them. There are numerous reasons why this happens. Some feel it takes too long to exercise; some individuals may have selected a time of the day to exercise that does not work for them (low energy level); or perhaps the wrong fitness program was developed for them. Of course, one of the key factors for success is goal setting. If unrealistic goals are selected, this can definitely be a de-motivator especially if the measurements used to monitor progress are not appropriate.

The following are some additional suggestions that can help you stay with your program and make it a success for you:

1. If you are new to working out, pick a program that is challenging but not overly taxing on your body. All too often people quit because they tire quickly, experience degrees of pain through stiffness or just simply find it too difficult. Pace yourself and gradually work up to higher levels of intensity as you build comfort.

2. Pick days and times that are convenient for you and try to stay with it. Having a steady routine is important to maintaining a good program.

3. Morning workouts, first thing, are the best. They clear your mind for the day making it more resilient for those tough hours at the office, school or day-to-day activities at home. Furthermore, it gets your heart pumping and maintains a greater caloric burn through the day. Working out in the evening can make it difficult to sleep since it does energize you. However, you need to pick a time that works best for you. If you have a higher level of energy at a different time during the day, this is probably the time you should try to work out. However, you will probably need to find a balance with work and/or school or other conflicting activities.

4. Sometimes working out with a partner can provide support, encouragement, individual competitiveness and even maintain commitment. Also, try doing a workout with members of your family, friends or even teammates. It not only provides a good bonding experience but enhances other activities as well.

5. When you start to work out, at least in terms of resistance (strength) training, try to focus on the major muscle groups like the shoulders, back, buttocks, legs, abs and chest. Since these muscles involve the largest muscle groups you will burn more calories using them and realize some shorter term, more immediate, positive results that will keep you energized. By working these larger muscle groups, you will also naturally work the smaller muscles like the arms.

6. Mix it up. Don't always do the same exercises or even the same order of exercises. This is not only good for constantly challenging the body but it also helps maintain interest and variety.

7. Remember some of the suggestions that were provided in earlier chapters: getting proper rest; maintaining hydration before, during and after exercise; and watching what you eat. All of these elements will provide you with

the energy you require to exercise and allow you to get the most enjoyment and benefit out of your workout.

8. Above all, be realistic with your expectations.

9. Practice your patience as it does take time!

TRAINING EXERCISES AND DRILLS

This chapter is the core of this book. It provides numerous training exercises and drills that can be utilized to help develop any type of full body workout you can imagine. It's simply a matter of applying your own creativity once you gain a comfort level with the exercises presented. If used properly, the sheer number of options and ideas presented with each exercise and drill will provide you with plenty of variety and challenge to last you a lifetime.

For each exercise in this chapter I will describe which muscles are impacted. You can refer back to the Anatomical Charts provided on page 36 and 37 to assist you with the specific location of the muscle referenced as it is important to understand what and how they are being worked. This will also help you with your ongoing and future development.

As you become more familiar with what follows, you will be able to modify specific programs and/or exercises to continually challenge your body. For example, a front lunge could be modified to include shoulder circles or another movement to engage multiple parts of the body together in one drill while also working on other important aspects such as coordination.

The variety of exercises (including stretching techniques) that follow, are consistent with the format of a suggested typical workout that I have outlined in this guide:

1. Warm up
2. Cardio
3. Resistance or strength training
   a) Lower Body - legs
   b) Upper Body – arms, chest, back
   c) Core – abs, obliques
4. Plyometrics
5. Martial Arts for Strength and Cardio
6. Stretching and Cool Down

Because Warm Up exercises tend not to change as much as other exercises even when fitness level increases, I have included a recommended number of repetitions that you should perform for each of those exercises. For all other exercises, suggested repetitions or timeframes are included where required to get you started. These will change over time based on your type of workout and your fitness level.

The earlier chapter which discussed proper form, specifically the section on Reps and Sets, was designed to provide initial guidance with the appropriate duration and/or number of repetitions and sets for the exercises you include in your program. There are also sample programs, in a later chapter, that provide repetitions, sets and durations to give you some additional guidance.

A number of exercises are considerably more challenging than others and they are identified accordingly. If you are new to physical fitness, I recommend that you do not try these until you have reached a higher level of fitness that allows you to tackle them without potentially injuring yourself.

The exercises are individually numbered so that they are easily found when you are working out. Also, the sample programs cross reference each exercise used to allow for quick reference if needed while you are working out.

Proper form is essential for getting the best results in a timely manner while avoiding potential injury. Since this is a "how to" guide, photographs and detailed explanations are included with each exercise and drill to help reinforce and maintain proper form. The photographs provide you with the basic direction you require, while the written explanations help to articulate the finer points. A larger font has been used for the exercise explanations so they are easier to read while you are working out.

Please note that props, or any other physical assistance that is sometimes utilized in other fitness periodicals for exercise pictures to show proper form, have NOT been used anywhere in this guide. My belief is that if an exercise cannot be properly shown without an aid I will not include it in this guide. Users of this book need to be assured that all of these exercises are possible, over time, with improved fitness levels and varying degrees of effort without being exposed to any undue risk of potential injury.

1. WARM UP

In the past, some schools of thought advocated that a workout should always begin with a good stretch. I tend to agree with this opinion provided the approach utilized is "dynamic" in nature and not "static". Static stretching will be incorporated into the workout format when we cover stretching and cooling down since the body will be warm and ready for this type of application.

Previously I mentioned that dynamic stretching is an approach that takes a joint and muscle through a wide Range of Motion (ROM) that is similar to exercise movements but does not involve any stress being applied to the muscles and joints. Since there is no stress involved, this becomes an excellent means to warm up the body, muscles and joints for a workout. Many of the techniques that follow in this section are dynamic types of stretching or movements.

Although the following techniques are provided for warm up purposes, many of them can also be very effective for your cool down. Some of the techniques included here, and in the upcoming Cool Down component, can also help you improve your balance.

#1 – Neck Rotations & Resistance

TARGET AREAS: Front & Rear Neck, Left & Right Neck

PROCEDURE: In a slow, wide circular motion, rotate your head 360 degrees in one direction 4-6 reps and then repeat the other direction to warm up your neck.

Once your neck is warmed up, I suggest you work the neck muscles. It has been included here because I believe it to be an important exercise (for posture at the very least and to help reduce the potential for injury) to complete before you do anything else.

All exercises can be performed in the sitting position (chair if you prefer) with your shoulders square to your body. I suggest you complete 10 reps for each of the four exercises to start with. For your front neck muscles (front flexion), place your hands on your forehead and press back with your hands while you slowly press forward towards the surface with your neck (see below).

To work your rear neck muscles (rear flexion), you essentially follow the same process as you did with the front except your hands are placed at the back of your head while you slowly press backward with your head as far as you can.

You can work your side neck muscles (left and right lateral flexion) by following the same process as above. The only difference is that you try to move your ear to your shoulder while resisting with your hand.

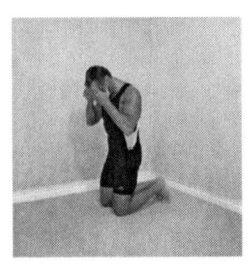

#2 – Wrist & Ankle Rotations

TARGET AREAS: Wrist, Ankle

PROCEDURE: Rotate your wrists in a **wide** circular motion one direction and repeat in the other direction (6-10 reps each direction). Perform the same motion with your ankles (ankles may feel a little awkward).

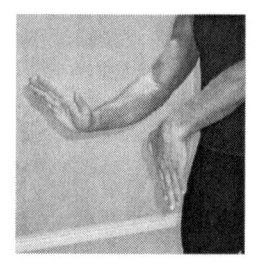

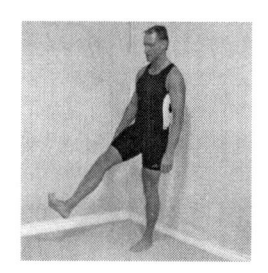

#3 – Shoulder Circles

TARGET MUSCLE(S): Delts, Rotator Cuff

PROCEDURE: In the erect position (knees slightly bent – not locked), keep your shoulders square and rotate either arm in a wide full circle. Your arm should be straight and the motion forward. Then perform the same motion backward with the same arm before moving to your other arm and repeating (Figure #1). When you complete each arm, repeat the motion with both arms together (forward, then backward) as shown in Figure #2. Complete 6-10 circles of each movement in each direction.

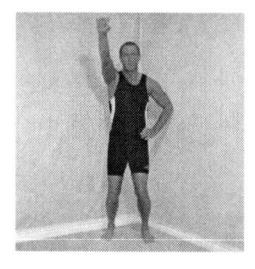

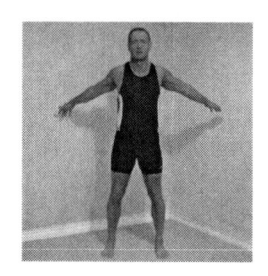

Figure #1   Figure #2

#4 – Integrated Shoulder

TARGET MUSCLE(S): Delts, Obliques

PROCEDURE: Lie on your back with your arms extended, level and flat on the surface as shown in Figure #1. Drag one arm across your body to the point where your palm is on top of your other palm while trying to keep your lower body (from the hip down) flat on the surface (Figure #2). Drag your hand back across your body slowly (take 3-6 seconds to come across) to the starting point as shown in Figure #1. Repeat this procedure on the opposite side and perform 6 reps on each side, alternating from side to side. It may take practice over many sessions to effectively reach over and touch the palm to the other palm.

Figure #1

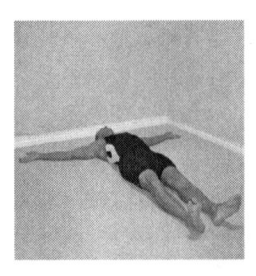

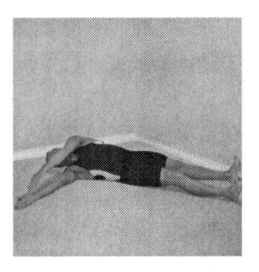

Figure #2

#5 – Hip Twist

TARGET MUSCLE(S): Hip Flexors, Obliques

PROCEDURE: Bend your knees slightly and keep your hands on your hips as shown below. While facing forward, rotate your hips only in a wide circular motion. Complete 6 reps in each direction.

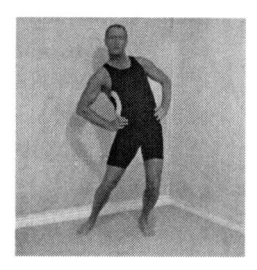

#6 – Integrated Torso

TARGET MUSCLE(S): Erector Spinae, Obliques, Abs

PROCEDURE: In the erect position, slightly bend your knees and extend your arms forward shoulder height. Make a fist with your hands and point your thumbs up to create a "sight of vision" as shown in Figure #1. While maintaining your extended arm position, slowly move one arm backside as far as possible (follow this arm by keeping your eye on the thumb and take 3-6 seconds to perform the full range of motion front to back) but ensure your front side "sight" does not move from the starting point (Figure #2). You might glance back periodically, or even use a mirror, to ensure your front arm has not moved. Repeat this movement up to 6 reps before moving to the other side.

Figure #1

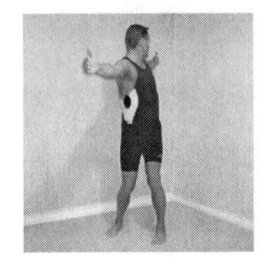

Figure #2

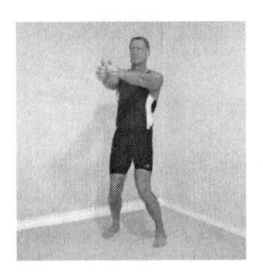

#7 – Circular Torso Rotation

TARGET MUSCLE(S): Abs, Obliques, Erector Spinae, Hamstrings

PROCEDURE: In the erect position, place your hands on your waist (or clasped behind your head). Rotate in a wide circular motion at your waist (try not to move your hips or bend your knees) so that your body extends as low to the front as possible (Figure #1), then to the side (Figure #2), then to the back (Figure #3) and finally to your opposite side. Complete the movement in one direction and then the other for 5-10 rotations in each direction.

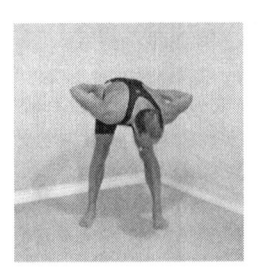

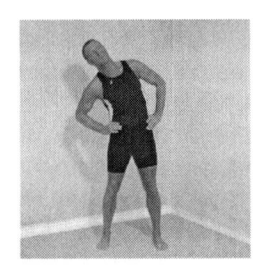

Figure #1

Figure #2

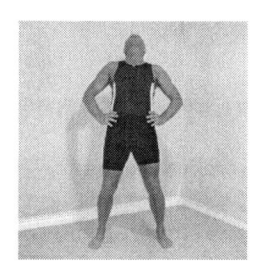

Figure #3

#8 – Toe Touch

TARGET MUSCLE(S): Abs, Obliques, Erector Spinae, Hamstrings, Glutes

PROCEDURE: Laterally extend your legs as wide as possible without bending your knees. Start with your arms extended shoulder height and do not bend your elbows (Figure #1). Bend down and twist at your waist while you reach to touch your toes, or as far as you can, with your fingertips as shown in Figure #2. Note that the arm you are not reaching with is extended above your shoulders as far as possible to enhance the stretch. Move back to the original starting position before reaching to the other side. Complete 6-10 reps each side.

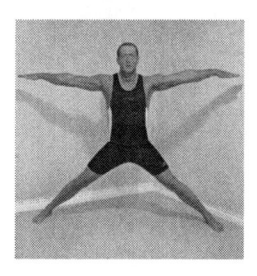

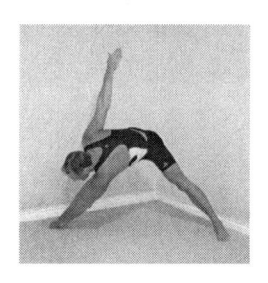

Figure #1   Figure #2

#9 - Leg Circles

TARGET MUSCLE(S): Glutes, Hip Flexors, Adductors

PROCEDURE: While in the erect position, bend your balancing knee (surface knee), and raise your other knee so it maintains a level position even with your waist. Keep your shoulders square with your body. Rotate the raised bent leg in a wide full circle **from side to side** (Figure #1). As your leg crosses the front of your body ensure your knee stays even with your waist line (Figure #2). Try not to shift your body to the side and stay facing forward (a mirror is always helpful to assist with form). This is a good exercise to practice balance but you may need to hold onto a chair until you gain comfort. Perform it in one direction 6-10 times (outside-in), and then the opposite (inside-out), before moving to the other leg and repeating both directional moves. Keep in mind the wider the circle the better for warming up the hip joint. Don't be surprised if you feel some "hip popping" during this exercise.

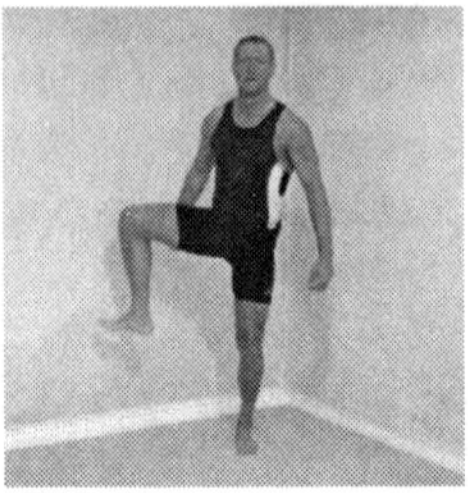

Figure #1

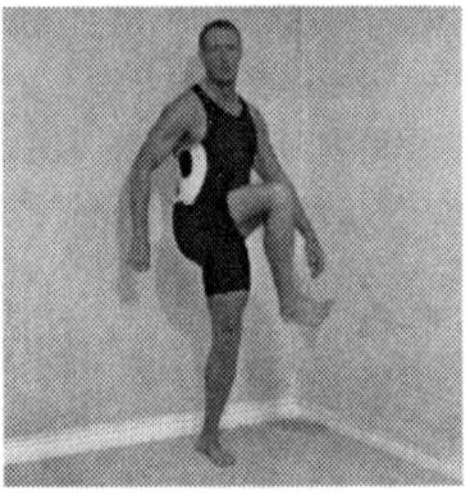

Figure #2

#10 – Integrated Hip (Advanced)

TARGET MUSCLE(S): Glutes, Hip Flexors, Adductors, Hamstrings, Obliques

PROCEDURE: While on your back, raise one of your legs so that the upper part of the leg (quad) is 90 degrees to your body with your knee bent. Try to keep your toes pointed up on your "surface leg" as this will enhance the stretch. Your arms remain extended and flat on the surface. While keeping your arms, back and shoulders pinned to the surface, shift your knee, as far as you can, over top of the leg that is flat on the surface (Figure #1). Hold for 3-6 seconds and switch to the other side following the same process. Complete up to 6 reps on each leg.

A similar version of this technique, that places focus on the glutes and hamstrings, involves extending your leg 90 degrees vertically while on your back. Push though your heel to maintain a straight leg while you move your leg across and as close to the floor as possible (Figure #2). At the lowest position, hold your leg for 3-6 seconds before switching to the other side. Repeat 6 reps for each leg.

A final version places focus on the adductors. The difference in approach from the previous exercise is that you move your extended leg outward as shown in Figure #3.

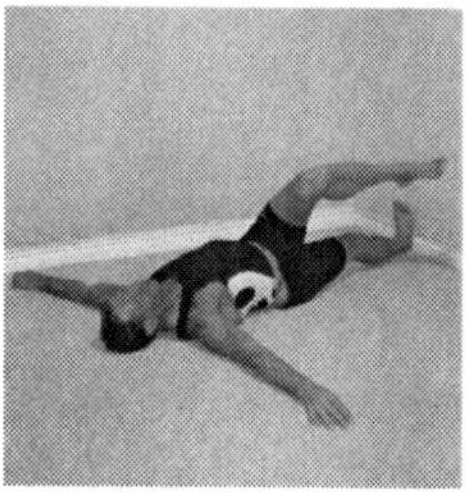

Figure #1

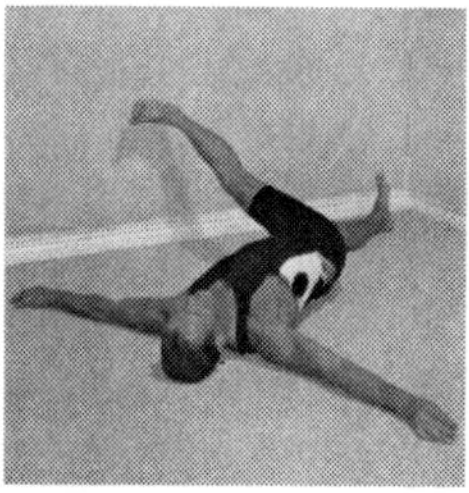

Figure #2

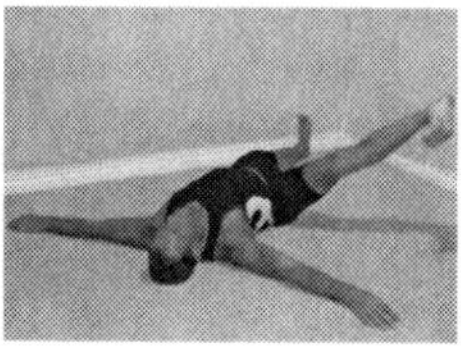

Figure #3

#11 – Cross Crawl

TARGET MUSCLE(S): Glutes, Hip Flexors, Calves, Abs, Obliques, Delts

PROCEDURE: While maintaining the erect position, face forward and bend one elbow 90 degrees while keeping your tricep level with the surface. Raise the knee opposite the bent elbow and cross it over to touch your elbow as you draw it inward as shown below. While raising your leg, tighten your abs and hold this position for a second before reversing the motion to the other side. You could perform this movement stepping forward or holding a stationary position. Perform 6-10 reps on each side.

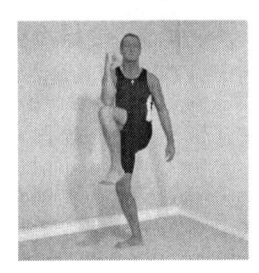

#12 – Extended Leg Kick

TARGET MUSCLE(S): Hamstrings, Hip Flexors, Glutes, Calves

PROCEDURE: In the erect position, keep your shoulders square with your body and your back leg extended behind you. Your front leg is bent. The arm that is on the same side as the back extended leg should be extended shoulder height and frontward as shown in Figure #1. Keep your leg extended while raising it forward to contact the palm of your extended hand (Figure #2) or as high as comfortably possible. Complete 6-10 reps on one leg before repeating with the other. With each rep, you could try to reach a little higher. Ensure your body remains upright and your leg fully extended by pushing through your heel.

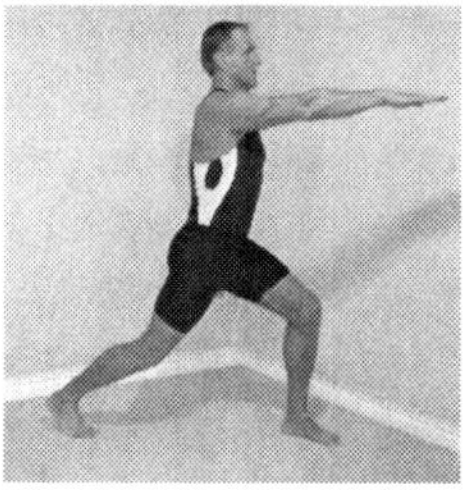

Figure #1 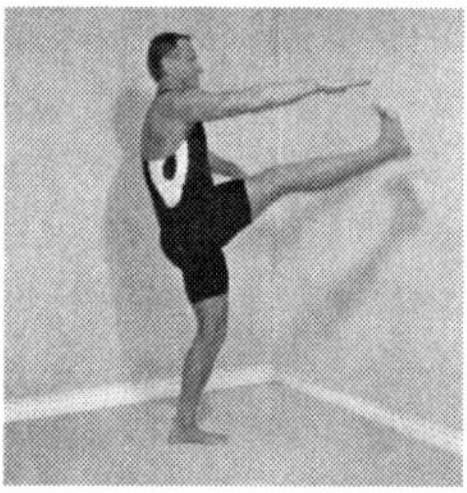   Figure #2

#13 – Knee Hug

TARGET MUSCLE(S): Glutes, Quads, Calves, Hip Flexors, Hamstrings, Abs

PROCEDURE: This is a high step warm up that involves a walking motion while staying on your toes. Raise your knee as high as possible bringing it into your chest, then wrap your arms around that leg and pull it tightly into your chest, holding it for a second while tightening your abs. Gently release your leg and lower it while stepping forward. Try to stay on your toes when stepping forward. Repeat the process using your other leg. Complete up to 6-10 reps on each leg at a slow pace.

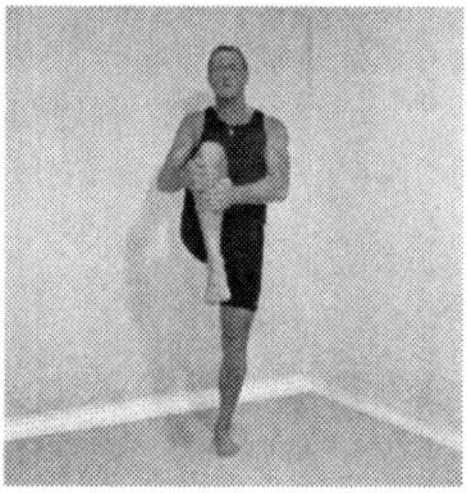

#14 – Hi Step Walk

TARGET MUSCLE(S): Glutes, Quads, Calves, Hip Flexors, Hamstrings

PROCEDURE: This is another high step warm up that involves walking while you stay on your toes. Raise your knees to your waist level, or higher, while swinging your arms as high as comfortable (higher the better) as you walk. Perform this motion slowly and complete 6-10 reps on each leg.

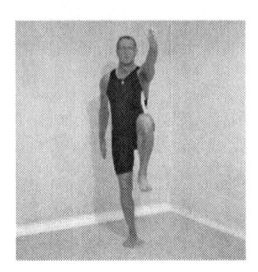

#15 – Spot Jogging

TARGET MUSCLE(S): Quads, Hip Flexors, Glutes, Hamstrings, Calves, Abs

PROCEDURE: A simple but potentially challenging warm up exercise that involves jogging on the spot for approximately 3-5 minutes, dependent on your level of fitness. Keep your body erect and stay on your toes while performing the exercise. Another variation of this exercise involves keeping your arms extended frontward, shoulder height without bending over (see below). This will bring your heart rate up more quickly.

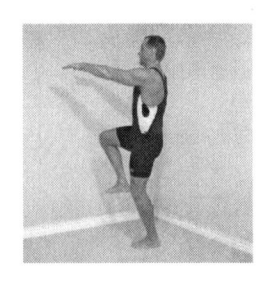

2. CARDIO OPTIONS

Cardiovascular training is an essential part of any physical fitness program. Sometimes this component of your training may be challenging to do because of time or other physical constraints. These challenges can be overcome with a little creativity.

The cardio drills provided in this section will help you complete this important part of your workout, considering your potential limitations in terms of available time and location. Obviously a good paced run, or swim, are always ideal for your cardiovascular development if suitable time, space and a facility are available. Some of the following drills may seem rather simple but once utilized you'll quickly realize how challenging they can be if you really apply yourself.

When you perform multiple sets of these drills you should rest between each set. The length of time you rest between sets should normally equal the duration of the actual set you just performed. You can modify the time somewhat depending on your level of fitness and how hard you are trying to push yourself on any given day. The key point is that you should select the appropriate amount of rest for yourself between sets so that you can maximize your effort for each set. You also want to ensure the rests are not too long so that you maintain your Target Heart Rate for the duration of the drill.

Suggested guidelines were provided in an earlier chapter for the length of cardiovascular training that should be included in a workout at the beginner, intermediate and advanced levels. Keep in mind that it may be challenging to maintain those levels when you first start out. To get you started, suggested timeframes and sets are included for each of the following cardio drills.

#16 – Stair Climb

TARGET MUSCLE(S): Calves, Quads, Glutes, Hamstrings

PROCEDURE: This is a straightforward yet challenging approach that does wonders for your cardiovascular and leg muscle development. Long continuous sets of stairs are ideal, like any hi-rise building or hotel, but any set of stairs will work like the ones you might have in your home.

If you are at the beginner level, start with 3-5 minutes of walking stairs versus running. As conditioning improves, try running stairs without stopping and while staying on your toes (5-10 minutes continuous is a great start) so it is less stressful on your knees and ankles while enhancing speed.

#17 – Spot Running

TARGET MUSCLE(S): Calves, Quads, Glutes, Hamstrings, Hip Flexors, Adductors

PROCEDURE: This drill is similar to Spot Jogging that was suggested for a warm up. The main difference involves pace, intensity and duration. There are some minor adjustments to form that you could also incorporate to increase intensity as your fitness level improves. One adjustment involves bringing your knees to hip level for the duration of the drill and another involves keeping your arms extended at shoulder level. Since this drill should be performed with high intensity, start with 3 sets of 10-20 seconds and increase this as fitness level improves. When you reach 6 sets of 45-60 seconds you might try combining it with other exercises and/or drills in this guide to enhance the exercise.

#18 – Hill Climb (High Step)

TARGET MUSCLE(S): Calves, Glutes, Quads, Hamstrings, Adductors, Hip Flexors

PROCEDURE: If hills are available, you might try running up hill for short periods of 10-15 seconds each. Raise your knees hip level while you run up hill and maintain arms extended forward. Walk down the hill for your "active rest" before beginning the next climb. Try 3 sets to start with and work up to 6. When you reach 6 sets increase duration by 5 seconds and return back to 3 sets. Continue to ramp up on duration and sets.

Another variation of this drill, for even more of a fat burn, involves the same execution except you go up the hill backwards.

#19 – Circuit Cycling

TARGET MUSCLE(S): Glutes, Quads, Calves, Hip Flexors, Hamstrings, Upper Body, Lower Body

PROCEDURE: If a bicycle or exercise bike are available, try cycling for 1-3 minutes (remember to maintain your Target Heart Rate) and stop to perform an upper body exercise (push ups); commence cycling for another 1-3 minutes and perform a core exercise (leg raises); and finally commence cycling again for another 1-3 minutes and conclude the entire set with a lower body exercise (lunges).

Start with 3 sets of this drill and build up to 6. When you reach 6 sets, go back to 3 sets and increase your duration on the bike or even add more exercises or reps performed, or any combination of the two.

Depending on your goals and your program, the exercises you select might be focused on the upper body, the lower body or strictly the core. This is also a good way to "mix" up your program, introduce variety and help maintain your interest level. You may also want to re-visit the sections involving Circuit Training and Interval Training to help with variations and approaches to this drill.

#20 – Circuit Jogging/Running/Climbing

TARGET MUSCLE(S): Glutes, Quads, Calves, Hamstrings, Adductors, Hip Flexors, Upper Body, Lower Body

PROCEDURE: Jog, run, climb stairs or hills as suggested in each of the previous drills but do this in combination. You may need to modify the duration of each drill slightly. The key is to "mix it up" and keep the body challenged. Try not to rest in between each individual drill until you complete a full set of what you have selected. Add sets and timeframes as your fitness and comfort level increases. I can assure you, you will be challenged and pleased with the cardio burn you receive.

#21 – Circuit & Interval Training

TARGET MUSCLE(S): Glutes, Quads, Calves, Hamstrings, Adductors, Hip Flexors, Upper Body, Lower Body

PROCEDURE: Simply follow the concepts and approaches provided earlier in the sections on Circuit and Interval Training (also refer to the chapter involving Sample Programs). These are great cardio options that can supplement or replace a workout and provide an intense fat burn.

3. RESISTANCE (STRENGTH) TRAINING

I emphasized previously that the cardio component of a physical fitness program is absolutely essential and should not be skipped when you exercise. That does not mean that a good physical fitness program should not include some form of resistance (strength) training. Resistance training is also an important ingredient of your fitness program that helps build, tone and maintain muscle mass. Even though everything in this fitness guide is based on utilizing your body weight alone, and not using external weights, you will still work your body and develop your muscles.

The exercises that are described below provide for a challenging full body workout. They are divided into **a. lower body,** like the quads, glutes and calves; **b. upper body** that includes the arms, chest and shoulders; **c. core and back** that includes the abs, waist and back.

When you execute the following exercises with proper form, and apply the approaches previously reviewed, you will find that you receive quite a challenging workout. You may even be pleasantly surprised to learn how aggressive your resistance training can actually be without the use of weights, or a fitness training facility. You will also find that this collection of full body exercises, combined with the wide array of methodologies you can apply, offer endless choices for workout challenges for a lifetime.

A. LOWER BODY EXERCISES

#22 – Front or Forward Lunge

TARGET MUSCLE(S): Quads, Glutes, Adductors

PROCEDURE: Keep your upper body erect, with your shoulders square and your hands on your waist. As best you can, fully extend one leg back while staying on your toes of that leg. It is important to keep your knee over the heel of your opposite leg (Figure #1) and maintain the forward position. In this position, the movement comes primarily from your outstretched back leg where it moves from a fully extended position to a bent knee that just barely touches the surface (follow a 3 count for this motion) as shown in Figure #2. Return to the original extended leg position, also following a 3 count.

As you become comfortable with this exercise you can increase the intensity by extending and maintaining your arms over your legs as shown in Figure #3 (you could even hold a small weight like a water bottle).

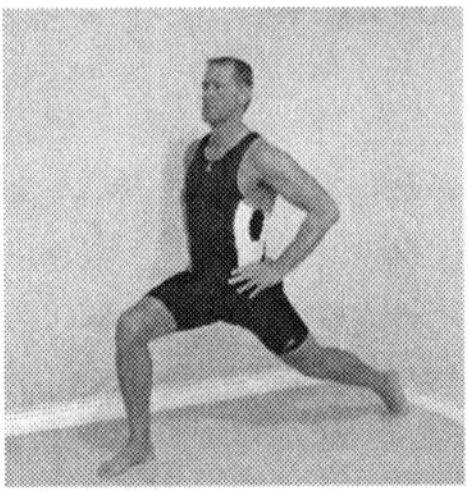

Figure #1 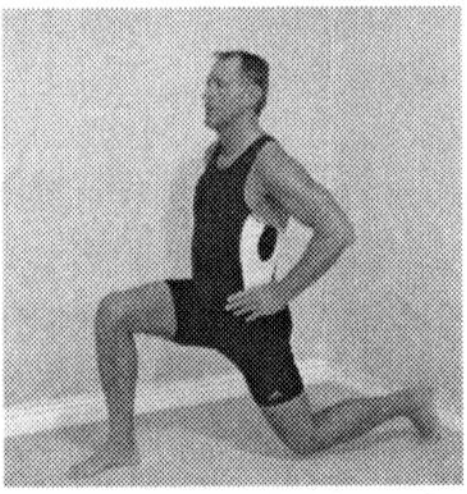   Figure #2

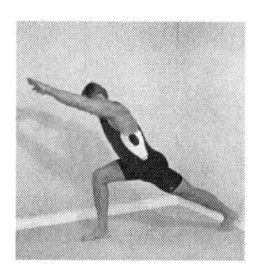

Figure #3

#23 - Extended Back Leg Lunge

TARGET MUSCLE(S): Quads, Glutes, Adductors

PROCEDURE: This is essentially the same procedure as the previous exercise except your front leg performs the majority of the up and down movement instead of the rear. You still maintain a 3 count each direction, as noted earlier. The exercise starts with both legs fully extended and the heel of your back leg does not touch the surface as shown in Figure #1. Your front leg then moves to a position where it is bent 90 degrees at the knee and positioned over your heel (Figure #2).

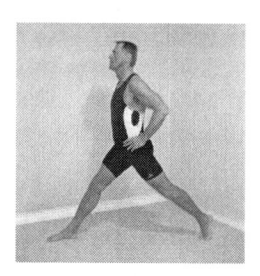

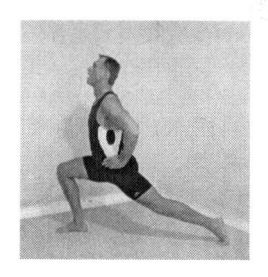

Figure #1   Figure #2

#24 – Rotating Lunge

TARGET MUSCLE(S): Quads, Glutes, Adductors

PROCEDURE: This is variation of the Front Lunge. The only difference is that you perform 1-5 reps on one leg and then switch to your other leg without rest. Once positioned, your feet do not move from their place as your front leg becomes the back and vice versa as you switch from side to side as shown below. Ensure you maintain lunge form as you pivot.

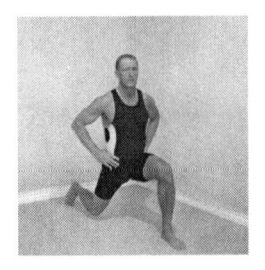

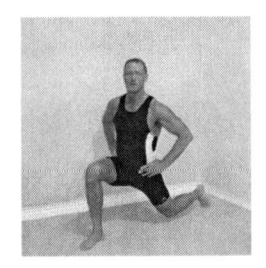

#25 – Chair - Front Split Lunge (Advanced)

TARGET MUSCLE(S): Quads, Glutes, Adductors

PROCEDURE: This is another variation of the Front Lunge that involves placing your front leg on a stable chair (Figure #1) while maintaining proper lunge form. Drop your back knee as far as possible towards the surface following a 3 count (Figure #2) and return to your starting position following the same count.

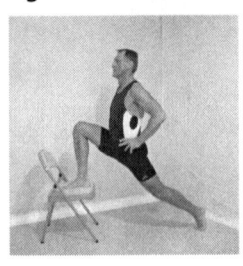

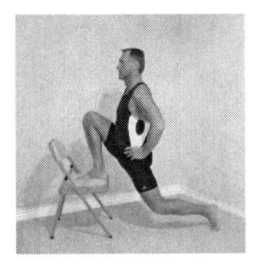

Figure #1   Figure #2

#26 – Chair - Back Split Lunge (Advanced)

TARGET MUSCLE(S): Glutes, Quads, Adductors

PROCEDURE: This exercise is a variation of the Front Split Lunge. The bent toes of your back leg are positioned on a stable chair (Figure #1). Ensure you maintain the Split Lunge form while the "floor" knee remains over your heel and the "chair" leg fully extended. Bend your back knee as far as possible to the surface following a 3 count (Figure #2) and return to your starting point. Do not rest your knee on the surface. Maintain an erect position with the upper body.

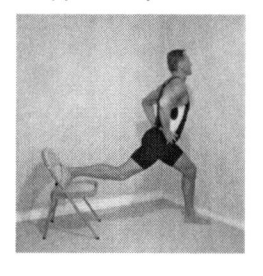

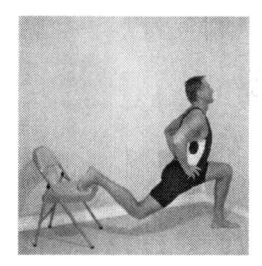

Figure #1   Figure #2

#27 – Walking Lunge

TARGET MUSCLE(S): Glutes, Quads, Adductors, Hip Flexors

PROCEDURE: In the lunge position (Figure #1), step forward as shown in Figure #2, and go into the lunge position with your opposite leg (Figure #3). Ensure that you maintain the knee over your heel and your upper body erect when lunging. Hold the lunge position for 2-3 seconds before you take your next lunge step.

Figure #1

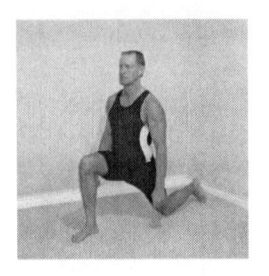

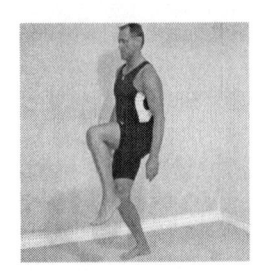

Figure #2

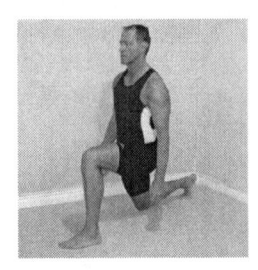

Figure #3

#28 – Standard Squat

TARGET MUSCLE(S): Quads, Glutes, Hamstrings, Calves

PROCEDURE: In the erect position, place your feet shoulder width apart and flat on the surface. Keep your pelvis tucked with your abs tight. Shoulders should be rolled back while you look forward, or slightly upward, to help maintain a straight back. Your arms could be extended forward shoulder height, however, do not lean forward or bend at the knees more than 90 degrees while squatting to 3 a count (Figure #1). Note the parallel position of the back relative to the shins. Always try to keep your knees over your ankles and your feet flat on the surface. Improved form would involve executing the exercise with your back towards a wall with your heels 75 mm (3 inches) away from the wall (Figure #2). This may take some practice.

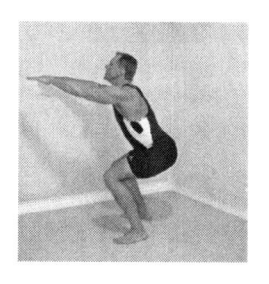

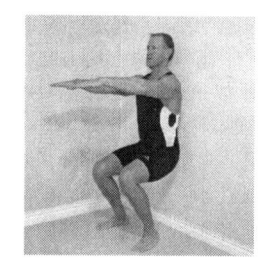

Figure #1   Figure #2

#29 – Wide Squat

TARGET MUSCLE(S): Adductors, Glutes, Quads, Hip Flexors, Hamstrings

PROCEDURE: This exercise is similar to the Standard Squat except you place your feet about 6 inches wider than your shoulders as shown below (find a comfortable position for your legs based on your level of flexibility). All other steps are the same as the Standard Squat.

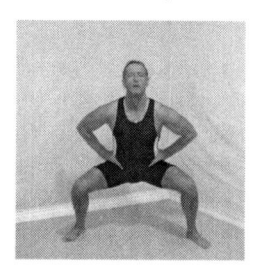

#30 – Side to Side Squat

TARGET MUSCLE(S): Adductors, Glutes, Quads, Calves, Hip Flexors, Hamstrings

PROCEDURE: In the Wide Squat stance, as shown in Figure #1, extend one of your legs laterally. Maintain a wide squat stance during the movement. The key is to try and move as far as possible laterally while extending your leg and maintaining a 90 degree bend with your opposite knee (Figure #2). Most of the movement will come from your hips while you maintain an erect, upper body position. Follow a 3 count each direction.

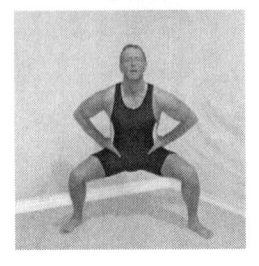

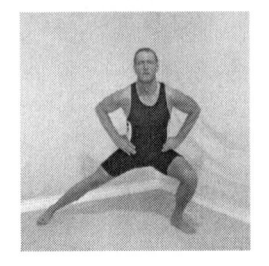

Figure #1   Figure #2

#31 – Chair Split Squat (Advanced)

TARGET MUSCLE(S): Hamstrings, Glutes, Quads, Hip Flexors, Adductors, Calves

PROCEDURE: This is a variation of the Wide Squat exercise where you place your heel on a stable chair, or bench, and extend your leg laterally (try to keep the toes of the "chair" leg pointed up) as shown in Figure #1. Maintain a Wide Squat form (the tendency is to bend over but try not to). Ideally, squat with your "surface" leg to a point where the knee is bent 90 degrees (Figure #2). Return to your starting position shown in Figure #1. Follow a 3 count for each up and down movement.

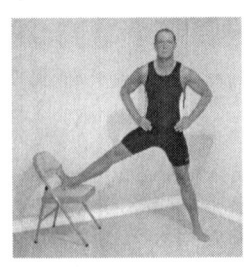

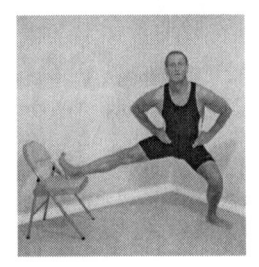

Figure #1   Figure #2

#32 – Low Squat Walk

TARGET MUSCLE(S): Glutes, Quads, Calves, Hamstrings, Hip Flexors, Adductors

PROCEDURE: While maintaining the Standard Squat position, walk forward. Lift your heels from the surface, as shown below, while you walk. Maintain a 90 degree bend with your knees and a straight back while you walk. It is easy to break this form, and if you do, it will reduce the load on your legs that is required to work them. Start with a distance of approximately 20 meters.

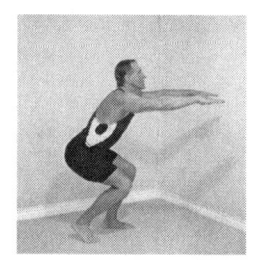

#33 – Duck Walk (Advanced)

TARGET MUSCLE(S): Glutes, Quads, Hip Flexors, Adductors

PROCEDURE: This is essentially the same as the Low Squat Walk. The only difference, and it is a key one, is that your feet remain level with the surface during the execution of the exercise. Clasp your hands behind your head while in the squat position (Figure #1). An option is to extend and maintain your arms shoulder height but most important is to keep your back straight. In the squat position, walk forward while stepping **flat footed** so that your feet remain level with the surface (Figure #2).

The greatest common mistake with this exercise is that individuals tend to come up on their toes while walking.

Avoid doing this as it reduces the load you want to place on the glutes. Also, try to avoid standing up and coming out of the squat position. Another temptation that should be avoided involves dropping your arms or placing them at your sides. Try walking approx. 10 meters to start.

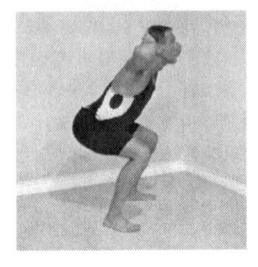

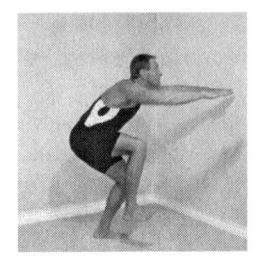

Figure #1

Figure #2

#34 – Adductor Leg Raise (Advanced)

TARGET MUSCLE(S): Hip Flexors, Adductors, Glutes

PROCEDURE: In the erect position extend your arms shoulder level and maintain fully extended legs. Alternately raise your legs from side to side as high as comfortably possible (ideally so that your toes touch your hands). With each rep, try to reach a little higher with your legs. Ensure your body remains upright and your legs fully extended by pushing through your heels.

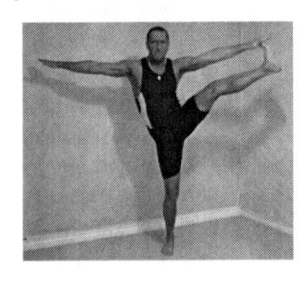

#35 – Stick Man Bend

TARGET MUSCLE(S): Glutes, Hip Flexors, Adductors, Obliques

PROCEDURE: In the erect position extend your arms shoulder height and your legs as wide as comfortably possible. Maintain fully extended arm and leg positions while you bend laterally at your waist and reach for your toes as shown below. Keep your abs tight while you alternate movement from side to side. Try not to bend over during the exercise.

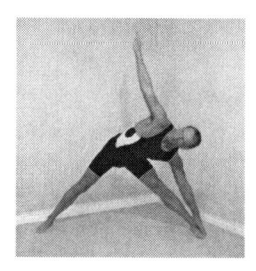

#36 – Scissors

TARGET MUSCLE(S): Glutes, Hip Flexors, Adductors

PROCEDURE: Lie on your back and extend your legs laterally as wide as possible (Figure #1). Maintain the extended vertical positioning of your legs so they are 90 degrees from your hips while you tuck your hands under your glutes for balance. Crisscross your legs as shown in Figure #2 and then spread them as wide as comfortably possible shown in Figure #1. Do not drop your legs and maintain full extension.

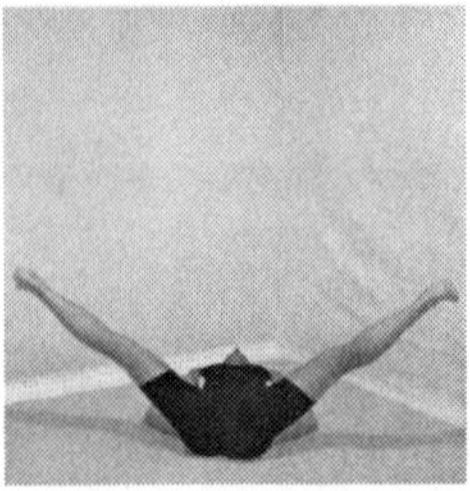

Figure #1   Figure #2

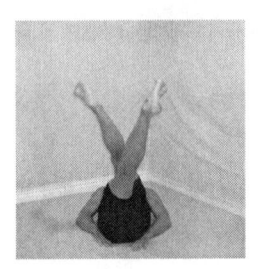

#37 – Bum Burner Bent Leg

TARGET MUSCLE(S): Hip Flexors, Glutes

PROCEDURE: Kneel down on your hands and knees as shown in Figure #1 (you might want to place a towel under your knees). Raise one of your legs laterally so that it is higher than your hip (Figure #2). Ensure your hip and knee joints maintain 90 degree angles as shown. Ensure your arms are fully extended, your hands remain flat on the surface and you look up to help keep your back straight. Complete all reps on one side before moving to the other and try not to rest when switching sides.

NOTE: For this Bum Burner exercise, and the straight leg version that follows, you can execute them with a 3 count up and a 3 count down or a relatively fast pace. I have found that both have different benefits. The slower count encourages muscle development while the faster pace helps with muscle toning and speed.

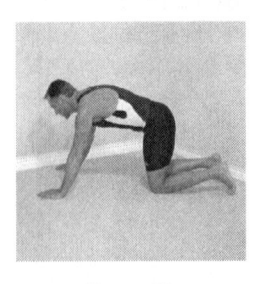

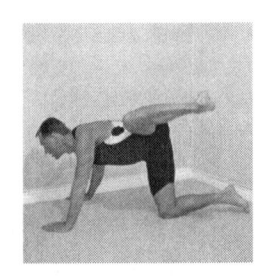

Figure #1   Figure #2

#38 – Bum Burner Extension

TARGET MUSCLE(S): Adductors, Glutes, Hip Flexors

PROCEDURE: This is the same approach as the Bum Burner Bent Leg except your leg is laterally extended and maintains a 90 degree angle to your body. To help keep your leg fully extended push through your heel. Raise your leg as high as possible and then lower it gently to the surface. Try not to drop your leg as this may create knee soreness and reduce the load (tension) you want to exert on your glutes.

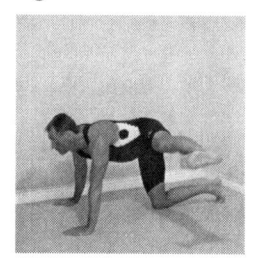

#39 – Bum Burner Kick

TARGET MUSCLE(S): Glutes, Hip Flexors, Hamstrings, Calves

PROCEDURE: This exercise is very similar to the Bum Burner Bent Leg. The only difference is that you maintain your leg at or above hip level (Figure #1) while you kick laterally (maintain a 90 degree angle as shown in Figure #2). Please note this is a quick "snap" kick from your knee and not from your hip.

Figure #1   Figure #2

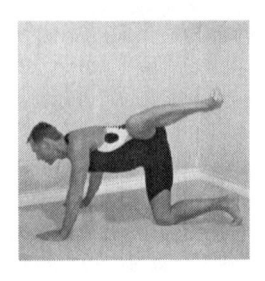

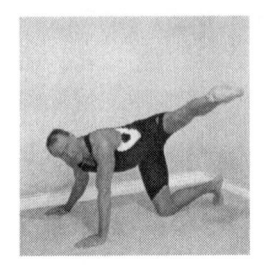

#40 – Bum Burner Hold

TARGET MUSCLE(S): Glutes, Hip Flexors

PROCEDURE: This isometric exercise starts the same as the Bum Burner Extension. The difference is that you maintain your fully extended lateral leg position while you rotate your ankle in a slow circular motion (see below). Ideally, try to keep your leg level with, or higher than, your hip. To make this exercise effective, try to avoid bending your leg – this in itself can be a challenge. Start with maintaining the position for approximately 5-10 seconds for each leg.

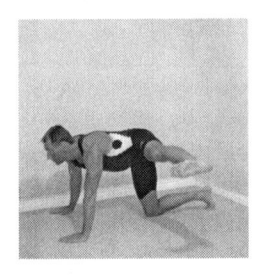

#41 – Bum Burner Circle

TARGET MUSCLE(S): Hip Flexors, Adductors, Glutes, Hamstrings

PROCEDURE: This exercise combines the majority of the previous bum burner exercises and uses the same form. Start on your hands and knees and fully extend your leg back off the floor while pushing through your heel (Figure #1). Lift your leg as high as possible while keeping it extended (Figure #2). Bring your leg forward and to the side while ensuring it stays level with, or higher than, your hip (Figure #3). Finally, lower your leg to your starting position without touching the surface as shown in Figure #4. All four movements should be performed in a continuous fluid motion. Try to maintain a wide circular motion during execution of the exercise to maximize the effect.

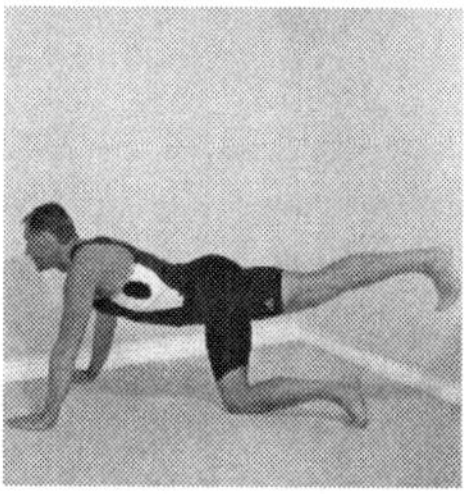

Figure #1

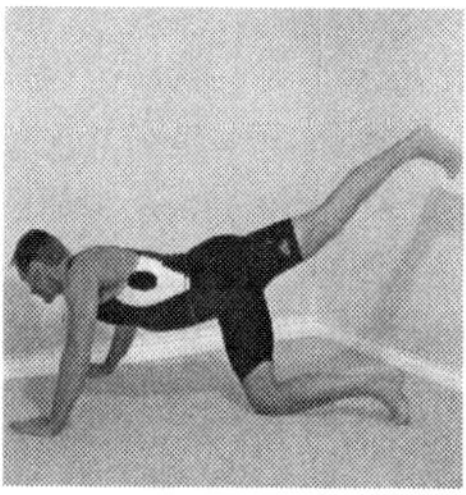

Figure #2

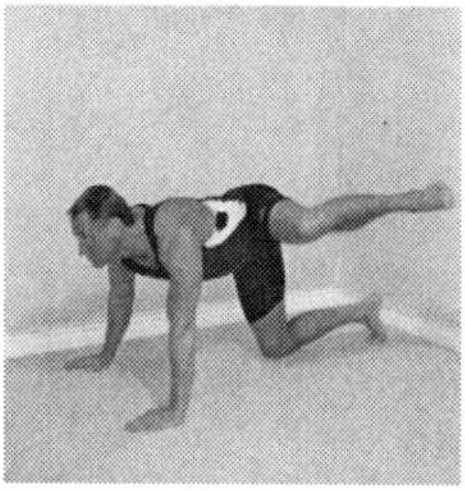

Figure #3

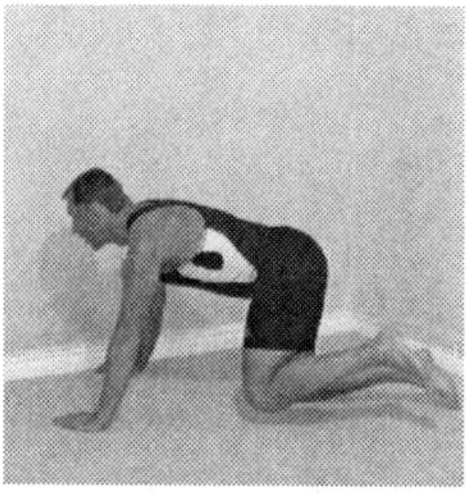

Figure #4

NOTE: To increase workout intensity, consider performing all five of the previous bum burner exercises one after the other in the order shown. An even greater challenge would involve performing all bum burner exercises, one after the other, without a break (super set).

#42 - Glute Buster

TARGET MUSCLE(S): Glutes

PROCEDURE: Lie face down on the floor with your arms extended shoulder level. Keep your arms pinned to the floor while you laterally extend one of your legs approximately 45 degrees (Figure #1). Lift your leg off the floor just slightly and hold it for a 3-6 count before lowering it back to the floor. Rest 2-3 seconds before repeating. Start with 6-10 reps each leg. This exercise tends to place primary focus on your glutes.

If you can raise both laterally extended legs as shown in Figure #2 (you may need to practice this version) it tends to place even more focus on your glutes and it also brings your erector spinae into play as well.

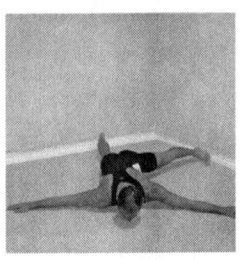

Figure#1

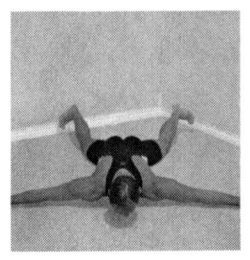

Figure #2

#43 – Toe Raise

TARGET AREAS: Calves, Achilles

PROCEDURE: This exercise involves standing on a stable chair, or stair, with your heels positioned below the level of the chair/stair. Your feet should be pointed forward, parallel and about 100mm (4 inches) apart (Figure #1). Lift your heels as high as possible to a 3 count before lowering to the same count.

A variation of this movement involves facing the wall and placing your hands against the wall just above your shoulders. Move your legs about a meter (3-4 feet) away from the wall while keeping your back straight and your pelvis tucked in. Your feet are still pointed forward and about 100mm (4 inches) apart. Try to position your heels flat on the floor and then raise them as high as possible following the same count. Take note that you can stretch your Achilles by bending one knee and alternating (Figure #2).

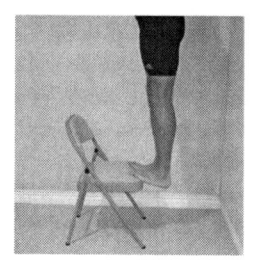

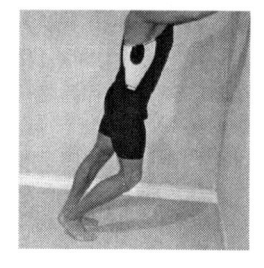

Figure #1

Figure #2

B. UPPER BODY EXERCISES

#44 - Standard Push Up

TARGET MUSCLE(S): Pecs, Delts, Triceps, Biceps

PROCEDURE: Lie face down (nose just touching the surface) and place your palms slightly wider than your shoulders with your fingers pointed forward. Your feet can be together or slightly apart. Your body maintains a prone position for the duration with only your palms, toes and nose ever touching the surface (Figure #1). Extend your arms as shown in Figure #2 (avoid locking your elbows) and then lower your body towards the surface. When you lower yourself, do not "bob" your head and try to keep it even with your shoulders (Figure #1). If this form is too challenging you can use your knees as the point of contact instead of your feet as shown in Figure #3 (keep knees together and your feet could touch the surface).

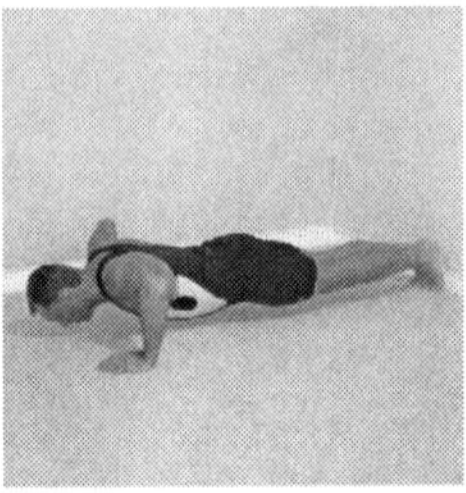

Figure #1

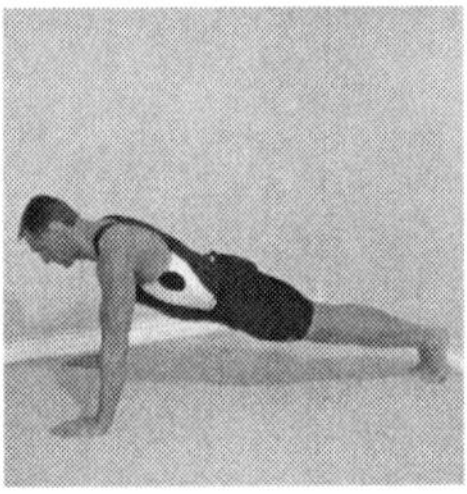

Figure #2

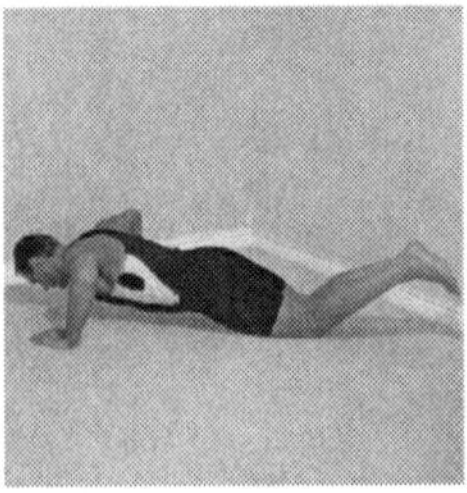

Figure #3

NOTE: The Standard Push Up provides the foundation for a variety of push up exercises that follow, hence the level of detail. Furthermore, if you do not have the strength to perform the push up exercises as described in this guide, you can use your knees for most of them, including the advanced ones.

#45 – Clap Push Up (Advanced)

TARGET MUSCLE(S): Pecs, Delts, Triceps, Biceps

PROCEDURE: All elements of form for this push up are the same as the Standard Push Up except that you clap your hands as you reach the extended arm position of the push up (see below). You can spread your legs to help with balance. After you clap your hands, ensure you drop to the surface in the proper push up form.

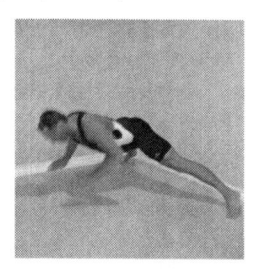

#46 - Tricep Push Up (Advanced)

TARGET MUSCLE(S): Triceps, Pecs, Delts

PROCEDURE: This exercise is very similar to the Standard Push Up. The only difference is that your hands and elbows are maintained at your sides as shown below. All of the movement comes from the triceps. Remember to maintain a prone position.

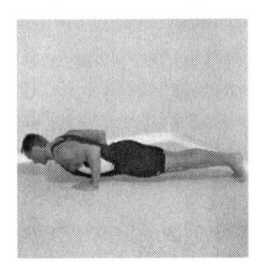

#47 – Leg Drive Push Up (Advanced)

TARGET MUSCLE(S): Pecs, Delts, Triceps, Biceps, Hip Flexors, Glutes

PROCEDURE: This is another push up variation that stems from the Standard Push Up. The challenge with this one is that as you lower your body towards the surface you bring your knee forward and to your side, as far as possible (Figure #1). Ideally, you should bring your knee up so that it touches your elbow (not your forearm). As you raise your body you extend your leg back to its original position (Figure #2). It will be challenging but try to maintain proper push up form.

A variation of this exercise involves bringing your leg into your chest as you raise your body (Figure #3). For a greater challenge, you could combine both variations shown in Figure #1 and #3 by alternating each type and alternating each side.

Figure #1

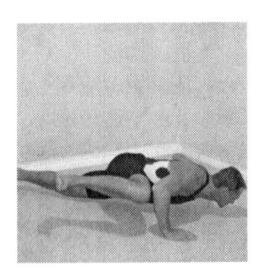

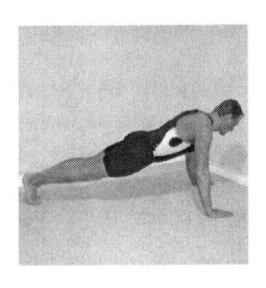

Figure #2

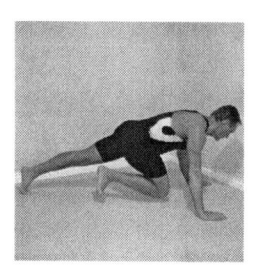

Figure #3

#48 - Tiger Eye Push Up (Advanced)

TARGET MUSCLE(S): Triceps, Delts

PROCEDURE: Form a triangle shape (Tiger Eye) with your palms flat on the surface (index fingers and thumbs together) while maintaining the proper push up form. Ensure the Tiger Eye is directly below your chest, keep your head up and spread your legs apart for balance (Figure #1). Lower your body so that your chest barely touches the Tiger Eye before extending your arms (Figure #2). Try to avoid resting your chest on your hands. Keep the up and down motion reasonably slow following a 2-3 count.

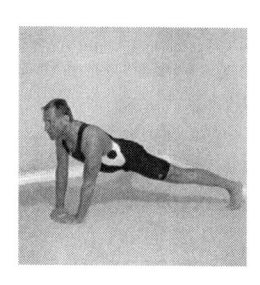

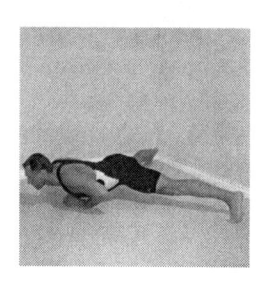

Figure #1   Figure #2

#49 - Shoulder Width Push Up

TARGET MUSCLE(S): Delts, Biceps, Forearm, Triceps

PROCEDURE: Follow the same format as the Standard Push Up. The one change is that your hands are placed wide enough so that you have 90 degree bends at your elbows and your fingers are pointed out. Your legs can be together or apart (your choice based on your comfort level).

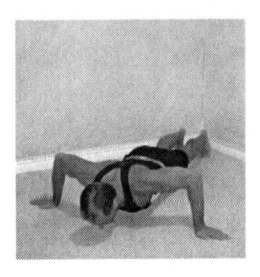

#50 – Perfect Push Up

TARGET MUSCLE(S): Pecs, Delts, Triceps, Biceps

PROCEDURE: Follow the Standard Push Up format again. For this exercise you can start with your arms fully extended and hold the position for a 3 count (Figure #1). Lower your body half way to the surface and hold that position for another 3 count (Figure #2). Lower your body to the surface (Figure #3), as low as you can without touching (hold to a 3 count), before reversing the entire sequence of three steps while returning to your starting position. This entire procedure is 1 repetition.

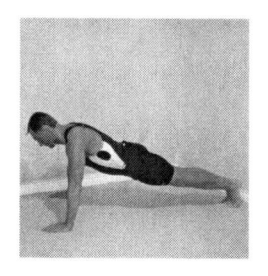

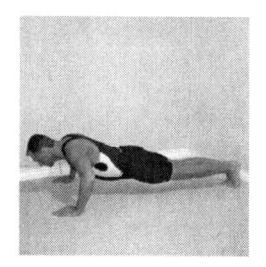

Figure #1

Figure #2

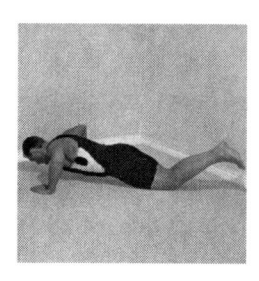

Figure #3

#51 - One Arm Push Up (Advanced)

TARGET MUSCLE(S): Triceps, Biceps, Delts

PROCEDURE: Follow the same general format as the Tiger Eye Push Up. For this exercise though, only one of your hands is positioned below the centre of your chest while the other remains behind your back (see below). Although I would not expect this exercise to be part of a typical workout, it is a test of strength and balance.

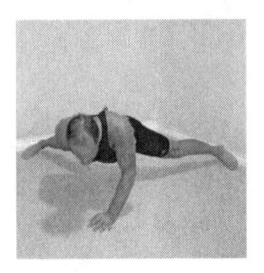

#52 - Scooping Push Up (Advanced)

TARGET MUSCLE(S): Delts, Pecs, Triceps, Biceps, Erector Spinae, Abs, Calves, Hamstrings, Adductors

PROCEDURE: Begin with the Yoga "downward facing" Dog Pose (extended arms and raised hips). Move your head and shoulders back as far as you can while your nose stays as close to the surface as possible to create your starting point (Figure #1). From the starting position, "drag" your nose forward as shown in Figure #2. As you extend your arms, look up as high as you can while arching your back (Figure #3). Note that your feet and palms remain the only contact points with the surface. Hold the extended position for a 2-3 count and reverse the movement to your starting point, dragging your nose slightly above the surface. This complete process equals one rep.

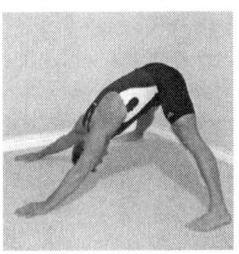

Figure #1

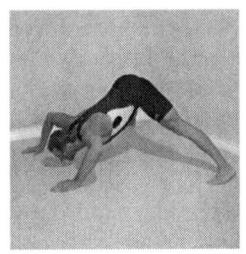

Figure #2

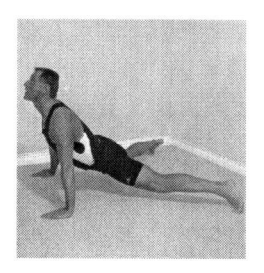

Figure #3

#53 – Side Push Up (Advanced)

TARGET MUSCLE(S): Delts, Triceps, Biceps, Obliques, Abs

PROCEDURE: Maintain a side plank position (straight body – no bending at your waist), extend one arm with your fingers pointing above your shoulders and place the other arm on your waist (Figure #1). Lower your body so your elbow is at a 90-130 degree position (Figure #2) before returning to the start.

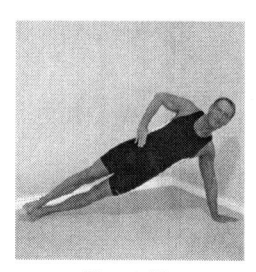

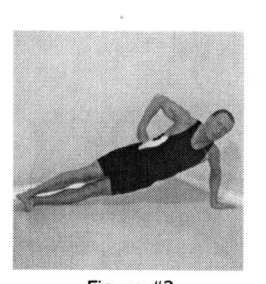

Figure #1   Figure #2

#54 – Side Twist Push Up (Advanced)

TARGET MUSCLE(S): Delts, Triceps, Biceps, Obliques, Abs

PROCEDURE: Maintain a side plank position and extend one arm above your shoulder as shown in Figure #1. Ensure your body remains "prone" while you shift to face down into a push up position as shown in Figure #2. It is one motion when you go from your side to the low face down position. Push back up into the position shown in Figure #1 to complete the rep.

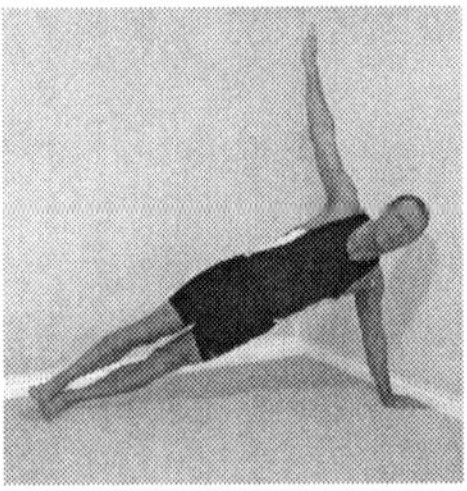

Figure #1 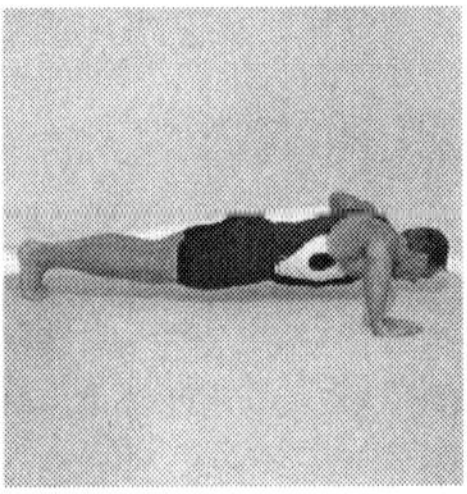   Figure #2

#55 – Dip

TARGET MUSCLE(S): Triceps, Delts, Pecs

PROCEDURE: Place your hands on the front edge of a solid chair or bench while sitting on the floor. Lift your body away from the chair so that it is just on the edge. Extend your arms but do not lock your elbows (Figure #1). Maintain fully extended legs for the duration of the exercise (push through your heels – toes pointed up). Lower your body so that your shoulders are level with your elbows **(not higher and especially not lower)** as shown in Figure #2. Perform both up and down motions following a 2-3 count (based on your comfort level).

The intensity of this exercise can be increased by placing both of your feet on another stable chair that is level with, or slightly higher than, the first chair (Figure #3).

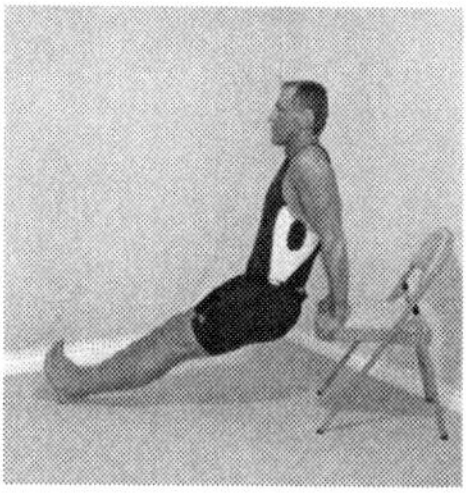

Figure #1

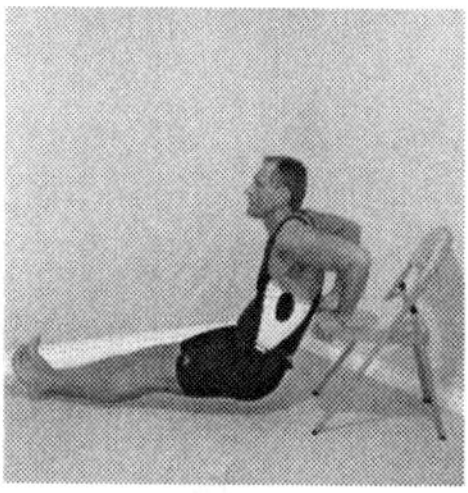

Figure #2

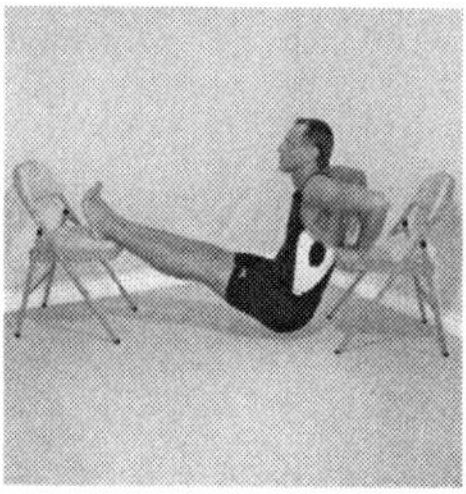

Figure #3

#56 - Arm Pull

TARGET MUSCLE(S): Pecs, Biceps, Delts

PROCEDURE: This exercise can be performed in the standing or kneeling position. Your shoulders should be square with your body and arms maintained at shoulder height. Bend your arms so that your hands are as close to your chest as comfortably possible. While maintaining your elbows at shoulder height pull back (twice) hard with your arms so that tension is felt in the front of your shoulders (anterior deltoids) and in the chest (pec) area (Figure #1). On the third "pull back" extend your arms while maintaining them at shoulder height (Figure #2).

Note: You can lean back in the "Seiza" position (a sitting, relaxed stretching posture used in karate) to stretch your quads while executing this exercise (see section on Stretching).

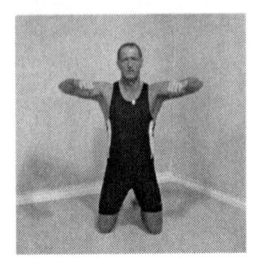

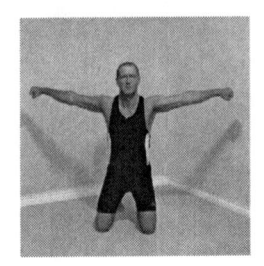

Figure #1

Figure #2

#57 – Tricep Dip (Advanced)

TARGET MUSCLE(S): Triceps, Delts, Abs, Erector Spinae

PROCEDURE: Place your hands at shoulder level (fingers pointed above your shoulders) and lift your body off the surface into the supine (straight) position (Figure #1). Keep your glutes flexed to help maintain the supine position. Bend your elbows about 90-130 degrees for each rep (Figure #2).

Suggestion: Perform Wrist Rotations as described in the Warm Up section before and after this exercise to reduce wrist tenderness.

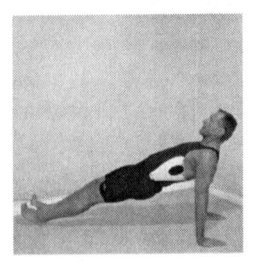

Figure #1

Figure #2

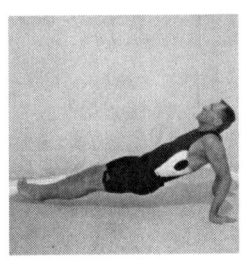

#58 – Wrist Rolls

TARGET AREAS: Forearm, Wrists

PROCEDURE: Use a bar or broom handle (or any similar item readily available) as shown below. Eventually you can try tying a rope with a small weight attached (water bottle) for additional resistance.

First place your forearms palm down on your legs while sitting (Figure #1) and roll the bar one direction and then the other. Then place your palms facing up (Figure #2) and perform the same rolling motion. Finally, hold a small handy weight, like a water bottle, with your palms facing inward and move your wrists up and down (Figure #3). Perform all three techniques in the order shown. Begin with 6-10 reps of each.

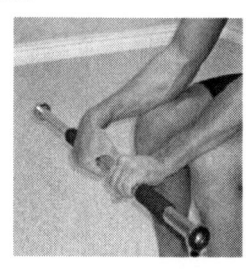

Figure #1

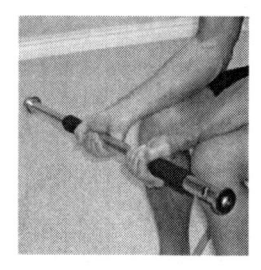

Figure #2

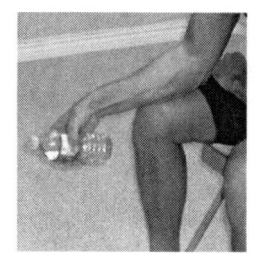

Figure #3

C. CORE & BACK EXERCISES

The Core is the focal point of your body in my opinion and consists of your rectus abdominis (abs) and your internal/external obliques (waist). I firmly believe the core is where the body derives its overall strength from and therefore it determines the level of performance you ultimately can achieve. This will be reinforced later in this guide when I introduce martial arts related exercises and drills for your workouts.

As I mentioned earlier, a healthy body and healthy mind go hand in hand. Similarly, I believe the core and back go hand in hand because a strong core will promote a stronger back. Because of my firm belief in the core, and its power, you will notice a considerable number of core focused exercises in this guide. If you adopt this same philosophy, especially if you are still in your younger years, I am convinced it will pay dividends as you get older, especially in terms of maintaining a healthy active lifestyle.

Keep in mind that when you are performing ab and waist exercises you must **keep your abs firm**. This will provide a greater workout for your waist and abs by enhancing the burn to those muscles and increasing the effectiveness of the exercise.

#59 – Standard Sit Up

TARGET MUSCLE(S): Abs, Obliques

PROCEDURE: Lie on your back with your knees bent and heels on the floor. Make a fist with your hands and maintain them at your ears. Keep your abs tight and bring your elbows to your knees (Figure #1). If you have difficulty keeping your legs in place while performing the exercise you could try placing them under something like a bed or a couch.

A variation of this exercise involves bringing your elbow up to your opposite knee as shown in Figure #2. This will create a twisting action that will assist with toning the waist (obliques).

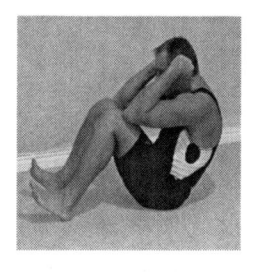

Figure #1 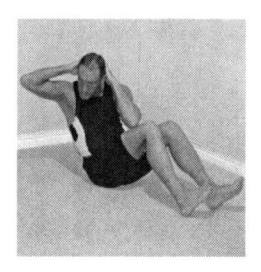   Figure #2

#60 – Leg Raise

TARGET MUSCLE(S): Abs

PROCEDURE: Lie on your back with your legs fully extended and tuck your hands slightly under your glutes while maintaining the position. Raise your head off the floor, if you are comfortable doing so, to help maintain tight abs. Raise your legs about 250-375mm (12-18 inches) off the surface (Figure #1). When lowering your legs do not let them touch the surface until completion of the reps you chose. Try to maintain a 3 count when raising and lowering your legs.

For an additional challenge, rest on your elbows while your hands are tucked under your glutes (Figure #2). The rest of the exercise remains the same. An even further challenge involves sitting upright with your hands flat on the surface at your knees (Figure #3) while raising your fully extended legs. The last option involves keeping your arms above your shoulders, slightly above the surface, while raising your extended legs (Figure #4). For a greater challenge involving any of the options noted, you could also raise your legs at a 45 degree angle from the surface.

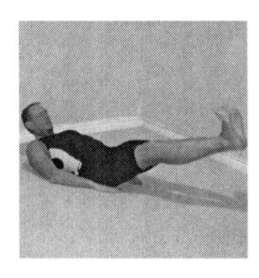

Figure #1

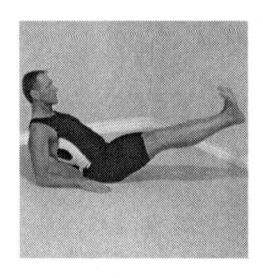

Figure #2

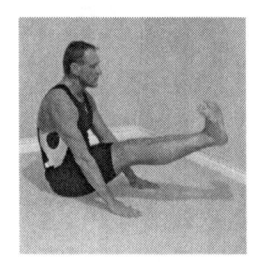

Figure #3

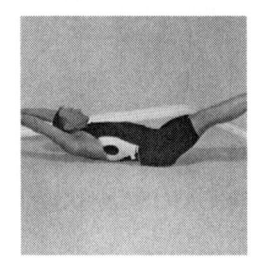

Figure #4

#61 – "V" and "O" Leg Raises (Advanced)

TARGET MUSCLE(S): Abs, Glutes

PROCEDURE: Start in the Leg Raise exercise position. For the "V" Leg Raise, maintain your legs at a 90 degree angle to one another or greater (Figure #1). All of the other steps in the exercise are the same as the Leg Raise. For a more intense version of this exercise, keep your legs spread/extended while raising them vertically as shown in Figure #2. A real challenge involves raising one leg while lowering the other.

The "O" version of this exercise is a variation of the "V" exercise. You not only maintain your legs at a 90 degree angle to one another, you also hold them at a 45 degree angle to the surface as shown in Figure #3. In this position, rotate your legs together in an opposite circular motion about 150-300mm (6-12 inches) in diameter. Perform an equal number of reps rotating the legs inward and then outward.

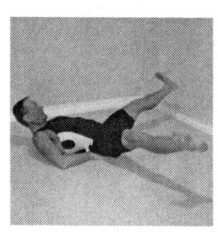

Figure #1

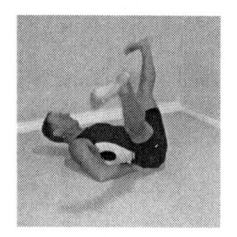

Figure #2

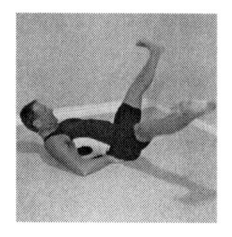

Figure #3

#62 – Leg Raise & Toe Touch

TARGET MUSCLE(S): Abs, Erector Spinae

PROCEDURE: This is a variation of the Leg Raise. Instead of tucking your hands under your glutes, fully extend your arms above your shoulders just slightly above the surface (Figure #1). Raise your arms and legs to a vertical position (keeping your arms/legs fully extended) and try to touch your toes as shown in Figure #2.

A more intense version of this exercise involves holding the position for a second, while you are touching your toes, and then reaching 50-100mm (2-4 inches) past your toes to complete the rep.

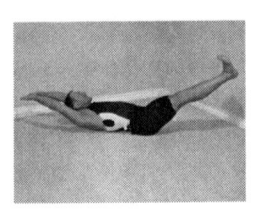

Figure #1

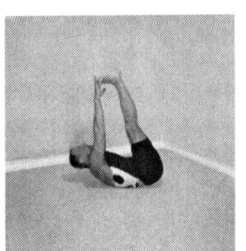

Figure #2

#63 – Punch Leg Raise

TARGET MUSCLE(S): Abs, Obliques

PROCEDURE: Sit on a chair, bench or on the surface. Either way, keep your legs off the surface and fully extended. While you hold your abs tight throw alternate hard punches (refer to the section on Martial Arts for Strength & Cardio for more information) as shown below in Figure #1. If you want to increase the intensity of this exercise, perform an upper cut punch or even a block as you twist (Figure #2).

This approach promotes a real burn for the abs and the obliques.

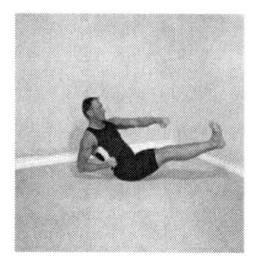

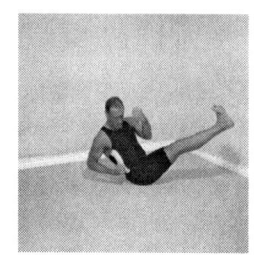

Figure #1

Figure #2

#64 - Vertical Leg Raise

TARGET MUSCLE(S): Abs, Erector Spinae

PROCEDURE: Lie down and extend your legs vertically (for this exercise you will need to push through your heels to maintain straight legs). Tuck your hands just slightly under your glutes for stability and rest your head on the floor (Figure #1). Raise your hips from the surface to elevate your legs as high as possible (Figure #2). Return to your starting position while ensuring you maintain vertical legs.

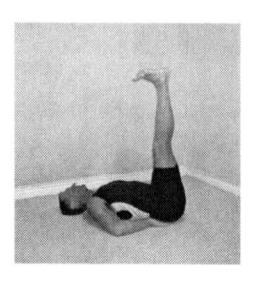

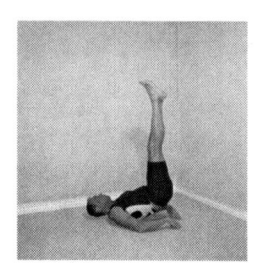

Figure #1

Figure #2

#65 – Leg Tuck

TARGET MUSCLE(S): Abs, Erector Spinae

PROCEDURE: Lean back in the sitting position with your legs extended and your hands placed behind you as shown in Figure #1. Lean forward while you bring your knees into your chest (Figure #2). Push out with your legs to return to your starting point. Perform both motions to a "3" count. An enhanced version of this exercise could involve performing a slow "riding a bicycle" motion while leaning back or even forward.

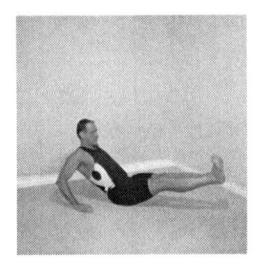

Figure #1

Figure #2

#66 – Push Back Leg Raise (Partner)

TARGET MUSCLE(S): Abs, Erector Spinae

PROCEDURE: This effective exercise requires a partner. Lie down on the surface with your legs extended. Hold onto the ankles of your partner that is standing at your head facing you (Figure #1).

Quickly raise your extended legs towards your partner (Figure #2). As your legs approach your partner he/she needs to push them back hard and fast from your feet. Your partner should not lean forward to reach for your legs but wait until they are close to them before pushing back. When your legs are pushed back, try to resist and prevent them from touching the surface.

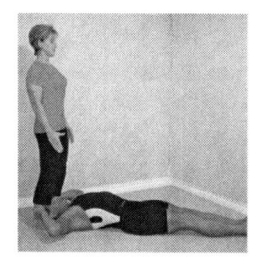

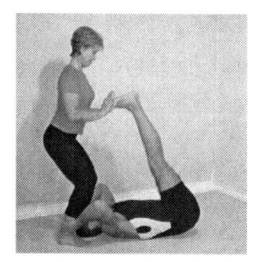

Figure #1

Figure #2

#67 – Scissor Raises (Vertical/Horizontal)

TARGET MUSCLE(S): Abs, Erector Spinae, Adductors

PROCEDURE: Lie on the floor with your legs extended. You can lie on your back or rest on your elbows. Tuck your hands under your glutes or extend your arms above your shoulders for a more intense exercise. Tighten your abs and maintain your legs about 250-375mm (12-18 inches) from the surface. Move your legs up and down in an alternating motion about 150-300mm (6-12 inches) each direction (Figure #1). Another version involves alternating your legs sideways as shown in Figure #2.

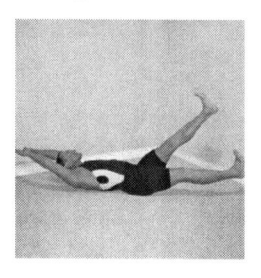

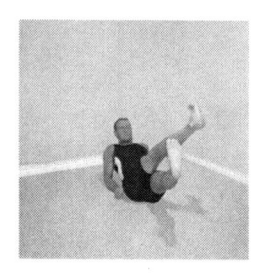

Figure #1

Figure #2

#68 – Seated Body Twist

TARGET MUSCLE(S): Abs, Obliques

PROCEDURE: Sit and maintain extended legs flat on the surface while you hold your upper body at a 45 degree angle (straight back) to your legs. There is a tendency to bend the legs but ensure you keep the full length of your leg on the surface. Extend both your arms shoulder height and clasp your hands in front of you (Figure #1). Maintain this position while you twist as far as you can one direction (your head follows your arms), to a 3 count, and then the opposite direction (Figure #2).

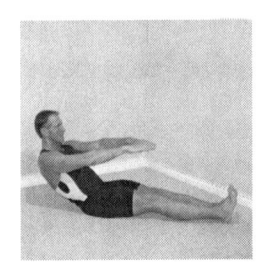

Figure #1   Figure #2

#69 – Bicycle

TARGET MUSCLE(S): Abs, Obliques

PROCEDURE: Lie on your back and extend one leg about 150-180mm (12-18 inches) above the surface while your other leg is drawn tightly into your body. You'll need to push through your heels to help maintain extended legs. Place your hands behind your head (or fists on your ears) and twist your body so that the elbow opposite the "drawn in" leg touches your knee as shown below. At the same time, try to bring your other elbow to the point where it barely touches the surface and hold this position for a count of 3. Continue this movement alternating from side to side and maintain tight abs for the duration. Keep your shoulders off the surface and promote a wide twisting action to increase effectiveness.

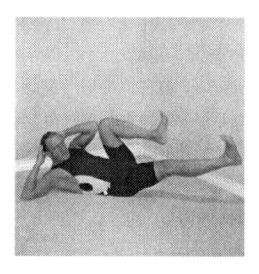

#70 – Side Crunch

TARGET MUSCLE(S): Obliques

PROCEDURE: Lie on your side with your knees bent at a 45 degree angle to your body. Extend your "floor side" arm above your head/shoulder and try to hold your shoulder off the surface while placing your opposite hand behind your head (Figure #1). Keep your abs tight while bending to the side in an effort to bring your elbow as close to your hip as possible (Figure #2). Execute this move following a 3 count each direction. Try to keep your back/hips perpendicular to the surface and do not lean back during execution.

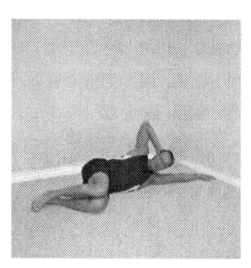

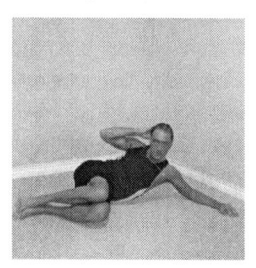

Figure #1   Figure #2

#71 – Knee Side Crunch (Advanced)

TARGET MUSCLE(S): Obliques, Abs

PROCEDURE: Lie on your side with your legs fully extended and off the surface. Rest on your elbow. Keep your pelvis tucked in and place your opposite hand behind your head (Figure #1). Bring your knees into your chest, following a 3 count, and try to touch your elbow to your hip (Figure #2). Extend your legs, following the same count, to return to your starting position. Note that your hips and your forearm are the only points of contact.

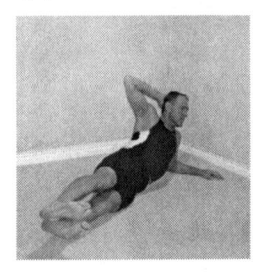

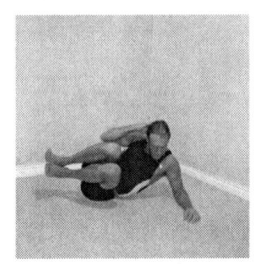

Figure #1   Figure #2

#72 – Standing Side Bend

TARGET MUSCLE(S): Obliques, Abs

PROCEDURE: In the erect position keep your shoulders square with your body. Bend to your side, reaching further each time with both arms (as high and as low as you can), following a 3 count (or reaches), as shown below. Repeat on the other side and continue alternating. Slightly bend your knee on the side you lean.

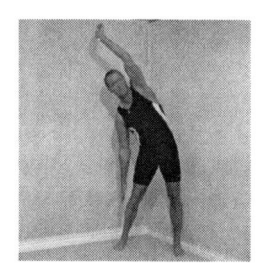

#73 – Boomerang (Advanced)

TARGET MUSCLE(S): Obliques

PROCEDURE: This is similar to the Side Push Up exercise except your arm remains extended through the performance of the exercise (ensure your elbow is slightly bent – not locked). The only part of your body that moves is your hips as they bend up (Figure #1) and down (Figure #2) to the extent possible (the greater the bend the better). When you move down, try to place your "floor side" leg (from the knee down) onto the surface. Try to keep your pelvis tucked in during execution. This exercise can take some practice to master but does provide excellent results.

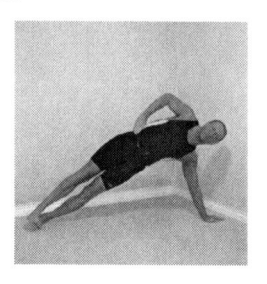

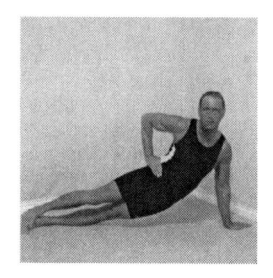

Figure #1   Figure #2

#74 – Ab Crunch

TARGET MUSCLE(S): Abs, Obliques, Erector Spinae

PROCEDURE: Lie on your back with your knees bent. Raise your arms above your head with hands clasped. Try to keep your shoulders/arms slightly above the surface (Figure #1). Tighten your abs and raise your body a further 100-150mm (4-6 inches) up from your starting position while you continue to look up (Figure #2). Try to avoid "bobbing" your head as it should remain stable with your body. Both the up and down motions should each be performed to a 3 count.

Another version of this exercise involves maintaining your legs in a vertical position, as shown in Figure #3. You could also alternate elbow movement to your knees as described in the 3 Way Ab Crunch exercise.

One variation of this exercise involves holding a handy light weight, like a water bottle (.5-1kg or 1-2 lbs), in your hands for the first exercise shown in Figure #2. Another approach involves keeping your arms extended at your side, and off the surface, until you have the strength to execute the other options.

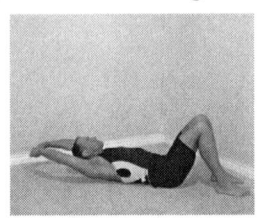

Figure #1

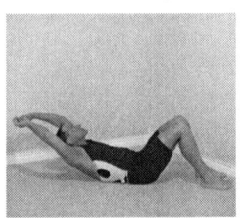

Figure #2

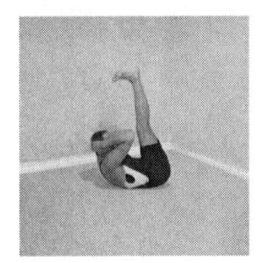

Figure #3

#75 – 3 Way Ab Crunch (Advanced)

TARGET MUSCLE(S): Abs, Obliques, Erector Spinae

PROCEDURE: Maintain your body at a 45 degree angle to the surface with your knees bent. Make a fist with your hands and hold them at your ears. Keep your abs tight during the execution of this exercise. In three successive motions, without leaning back more than 45 degrees in between each movement; 1) bring one elbow as close to your opposite knee as possible (Figure #1); 2) bring both elbows to the knees (Figure #2); and 3) bring your opposite elbow to the other knee. Each motion should be performed to a 3 count.

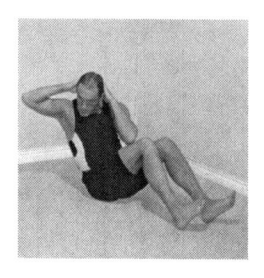

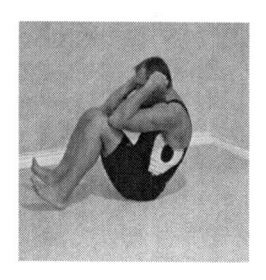

Figure #1   Figure #2

#76 – Turbo Twist

TARGET MUSCLE(S): Abs, Obliques, Erector Spinae

PROCEDURE: Stand with your knees slightly bent and raise your arms/elbows shoulder height while maintaining a 90 degree bend at your elbows (see below). Twist as far as possible in each direction without losing your form and maintain a tight core at all times. Start off slow initially, but ramp up during the exercise to perform it as fast as possible for the selected time or reps.

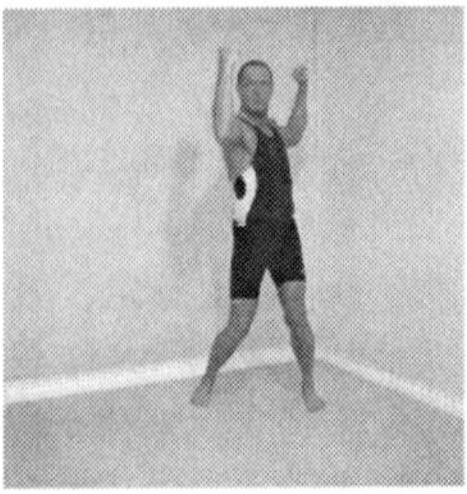

#77 – Oblique Reach

TARGET MUSCLE(S): Abs, Obliques

PROCEDURE: Lie down and maintain both legs fully extended (one about 30 degrees from the surface and the other vertical). Extend your arms shoulder level, maintain tight abs and keep your head slightly off the surface (Figure #1). Rise up to touch the outside ankle of your vertical leg, or as close as possible, with your opposite hand as shown in Figure #2. Hold for a 3 count before slowly lowering your body (Figure #1).

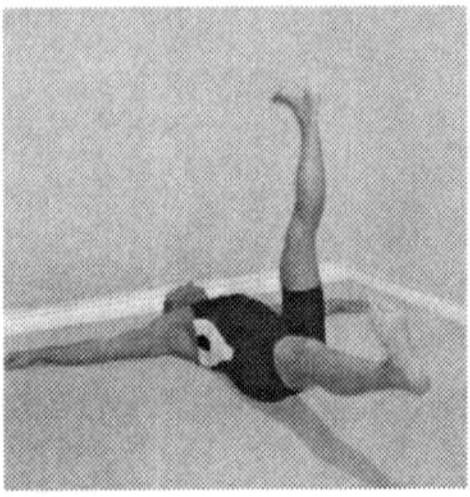

Figure #1

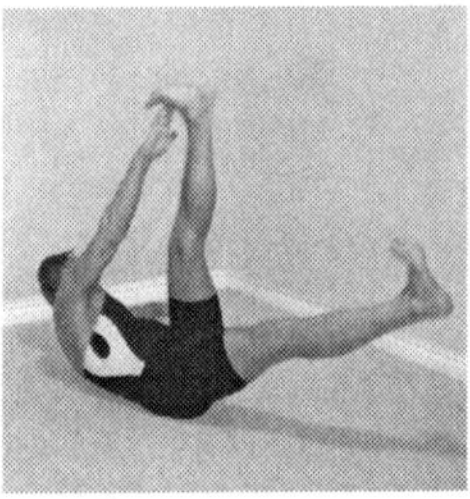

Figure #2

#78 - Back Challenge

TARGET MUSCLE(S): Erector Spinae, Abs

PROCEDURE: Lie face down on the surface with your arms extended shoulder level. Keep your arms pinned to the floor while you extend both legs at approximately 30-45 degrees from your body (the wider the better) as shown below. Lift both legs off the surface and hold them for a 3-6 count before lowering them. Rest 2-3 seconds before repeating. Start with 6-10 reps.

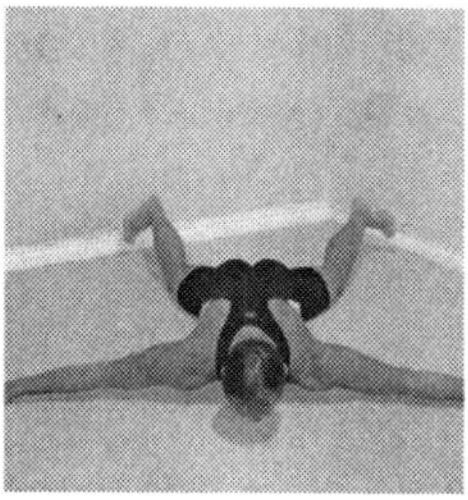

#79 - Superman

TARGET MUSCLE(S): Erector Spinae, Abs

PROCEDURE: Lie face down on the floor and maintain extended arms and legs off the floor as shown in Figure #1. You can also perform this exercise using a ball, if available, or even a stable chair or bench to help practice balance (Figure #2).

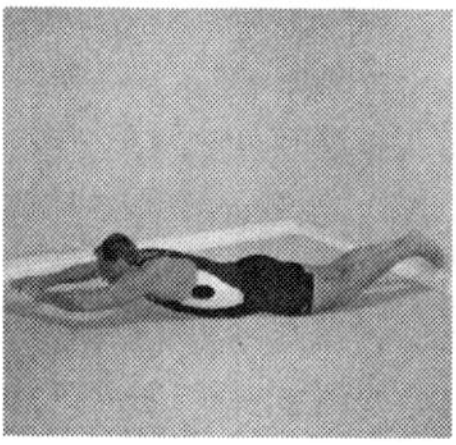

Figure #1 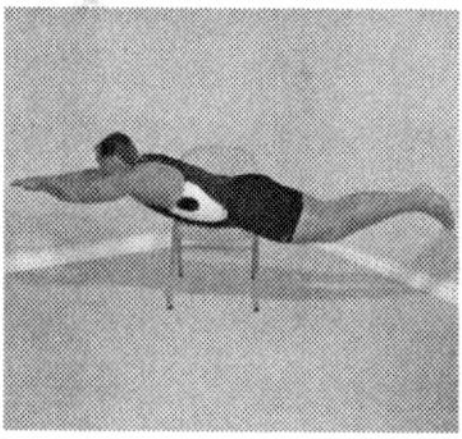   Figure #2

#80 – Superman Twist (Advanced)

TARGET MUSCLE(S): Erector Spinae, Abs, Obliques

PROCEDURE: Lie face down with your hands clasped behind your head. Tuck your feet under something, like a chair, for support. Raise your upper body from the surface and look up (this will help elevate your body) as shown in Figure #1. Once your body is as high as you can raise it, twist one direction and then the other (Figure #2). Return to the surface and repeat. You may need to start with twisting to one side only before repeating, or simply raising up, until you have the strength to perform both twists.

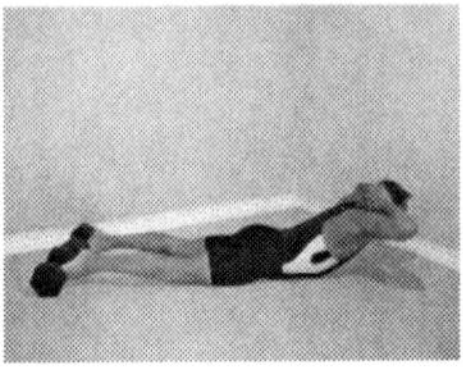

Figure #1 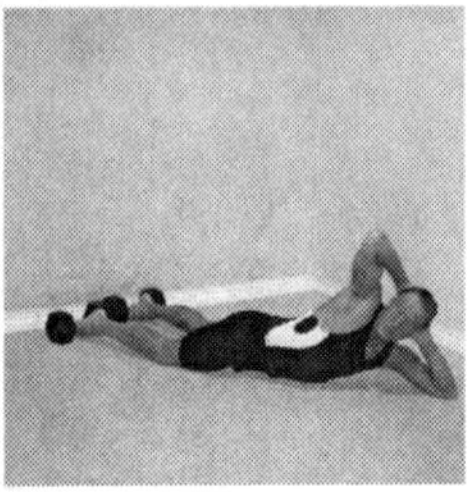   Figure #2

#81 – Reverse Superman

TARGET MUSCLE(S): Abs, Obliques

PROCEDURE: Lie down with your arms and legs fully extended. Raise them 50-150mm (2-6 inches) off the surface and maintain this position for 3-6 seconds as shown below (this is one rep). Note the extended legs, the upper body and neck remain isolated. You could add a variation to this exercise and twist with your hands behind your head (or fists held at your ears), like the previous exercise, to engage the obliques.

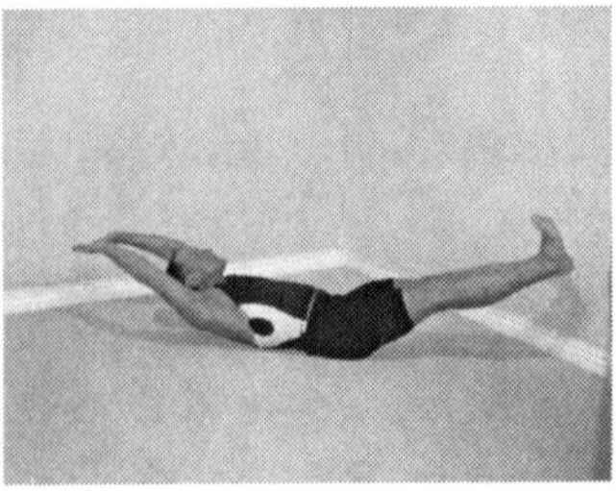

#82 – Oblique Crunch

TARGET MUSCLE(S): Obliques, Abs

PROCEDURE: In the sit up position, place one knee over the other and keep them together tightly. Clasp your hands behind your head but do not pull on your neck. Maintain tight abs with your shoulders off the surface for the duration of the exercise – this is important. Bring your elbow to the knee of your opposite leg that is crossed over as shown below. When you lower your body, keep your shoulders slightly off the surface. This is a fast paced exercise which involves a "crunch and twist" designed to keep tension on your abs and obliques.

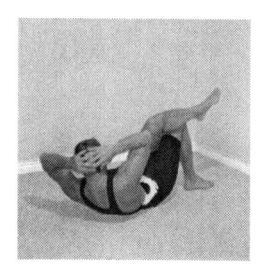

#83 – Vertical Oblique Twist

TARGET MUSCLE(S): Obliques, Abs, Erector Spinae

PROCEDURE: Lie flat with your arms extended shoulder height and maintain extended legs (Figure #1). Pivot from your hips, side to side, and try to touch your feet to the surface. Notice that your arms and shoulders remain flat on the surface (Figure #2). A variation of this exercise involves full vertical extension of your arms and your legs. Pivot your legs the same way as you did in the previous exercise. The slight variation is that this time you reach in the opposite direction with your arms that are clasped together as shown in Figure #3. This is also a great exercise for practicing balance.

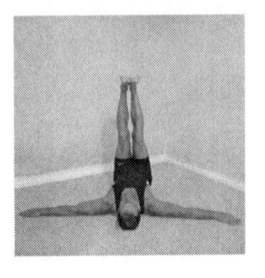

Figure #1

Figure #2

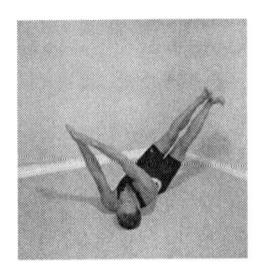

Figure #3

#84 – Prone & Supine

TARGET MUSCLE(S): Abs, Erector Spinae, Hamstrings, Glutes

PROCEDURE: Lie face down and maintain a "straight plank" (prone) position with tight abs while resting on your elbows and toes (Figure #1). Hold this isometric position for a selected time (try 10 seconds to start with and work up over time).

A second and advanced variation of this exercise involves maintaining the supine position (Figure #2). Ensure that your glutes and lower back remain tight during the exercise.

An advanced modification of this exercise involves fully extending your legs, while maintaining the form previously described, and raising them in an alternating manner while maintaining the supine position (Figure #3). A final approach involves the prone position where you extend your leg laterally, 45 degrees from your body, and alternate from side to side, as shown in Figure #4.

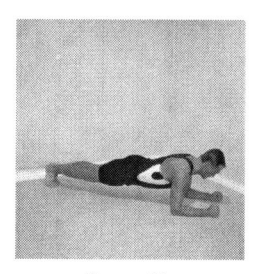

Figure #1

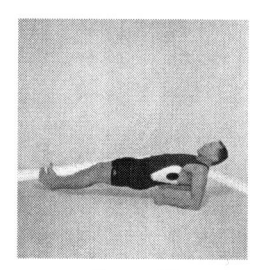

Figure #2

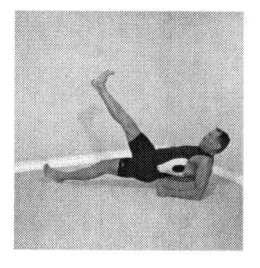

Figure #3

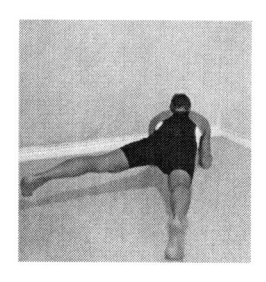

Figure #4

#85 - 3 Way Ab Plank

TARGET MUSCLE(S): Abs, Obliques, Erector Spinae

PROCEDURE: This is essentially the same exercise as the Prone except you start on your side, resting on your elbow (Figure #1) and hold the position for 3 seconds; then move to the face down position (Figure #2) and hold again for 3 seconds; and lastly move to the other side, similar to Figure #1, to complete your rep. Continue by reversing direction for the reps you selected.

Figure #1

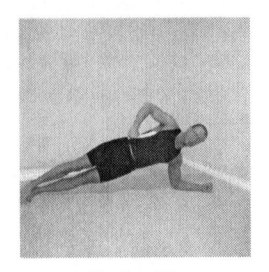

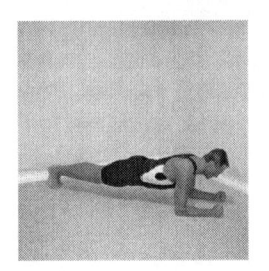

Figure #2

4. PLYOMETRICS

Plyometric exercises are special training exercises that help provide powerful explosive muscle response that not only enhance the intensity of a workout but can also assist with developing speed, agility, quickness and coordination. Typically they involve some form of jumping, hopping or leaping. As a result, they provide a high level of intensity that can help enhance a cardio workout if utilized properly. Although plyometrics are great for an exercise program, and increasing your caloric burn, they should be used with care.

Since plyometrics are generally high impact exercises they should only be incorporated into your program once you are physically well conditioned. Due to the nature of plyometrics, I strongly recommend you use them to add variety and challenge to your program but do not use them excessively.

Before you include plyometric exercises in your fitness program, you should be well versed with proper and safe landing techniques. Always land with your knees slightly bent, while staying on your toes, and then roll back onto your heels. When you land you should also try to avoid any twisting or sideways motion at the knee joint. In an article called "Plyometric Exercises – Using Plyometric Exercises to Build Speed and Power", About.com, December 8, 2008, Elizabeth Quinn included the following very good plyometric safety tips:

1. Recommended only for athletes that are well conditioned

2. For individuals that have high levels of strength

3. Warm up thoroughly before doing
4. Start slowly with small jumps and gradually build up
5. Land softly to absorb the shock
6. Allow plenty of rest between plyometric workouts
7. Stop immediately if you feel joint pain
8. Pay attention to Injury Warning Signs
9. Use footwear with plenty of cushioning
10. Perform the exercises on soft or cushioned surfaces like grass

#86 – Jumping Jacks

TARGET MUSCLE(S): Delts, Glutes, Calves, Quads, Hip Flexors, Hamstrings, Adductors

PROCEDURE: In the erect position place your arms at your side with your legs together (Figure #1). While jumping slightly off the floor, with your knees bent, spread your legs wide apart and bring your arms above your head as shown in Figure #2 (try to keep your arms straight at all times to increase the load on your shoulders). Also, try to stay on your toes (balls of your feet), and keep your knees bent, to help reduce the impact to your knees and ankles.

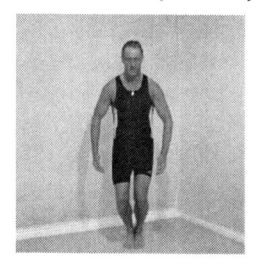

Figure #1   Figure #2

#87 – Double Up Jumping Jacks (Advanced)

TARGET MUSCLE(S): Quads, Glutes, Hip Flexors, Adductors, Hamstrings, Calves, Delts

PROCEDURE: This exercise is the same as Jumping Jacks but is designed to be a more advanced technique to help develop coordination and speed. The difference is that you start in the "legs apart" position instead of legs together (Figure #2 above). When you jump up, you bring your legs together and very quickly spread them apart again before landing on the balls of your feet. This will take practice, coordination and focus to master.

#88 – Split Jumping Jacks – Reverse Direction

TARGET MUSCLE(S): Quads, Glutes, Calves, Adductors, Hamstrings, Hip Flexors, Delts

PROCEDURE: This is another exercise that is consistent with Jumping Jacks but has a slight twist that will challenge your coordination. You begin with completing a rep of the typical Jumping Jack shown previously. Instead of beginning a second similar rep when you bring your feet together, perform the next reps with each of your arms and legs moving forward and backward in a scissors motion as shown below. This entire sequence (sideways/forward/backward) completes one rep. Return to the "legs together" position, as in Figure #1 of the Jumping Jacks exercise, to start the next rep.

This movement will require some practice to perfect but does help to develop coordination.

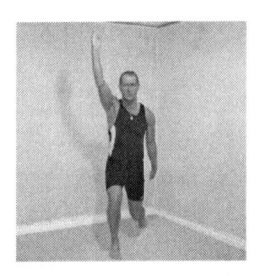

#89 – Jump Squat

TARGET MUSCLE(S): Glutes, Quads, Calves, Hamstrings, Hip Flexors, Adductors

PROCEDURE: In the Standard Squat position, place your arms just in front of you, or at your sides, and your feet flat on the surface (Figure #1). Leap up as high as you can while fully extending your arms above your shoulders (Figure #2).

Return to a proper squat position and hold for a second before performing another rep. Maintain a straight back and proper squat form when landing.

If space permits, a variation of this drill involves leaping forward instead of straight up. If you leap forward, start with a distance of about 20 meters for one set and gradually add to your jumping distance as your fitness level improves.

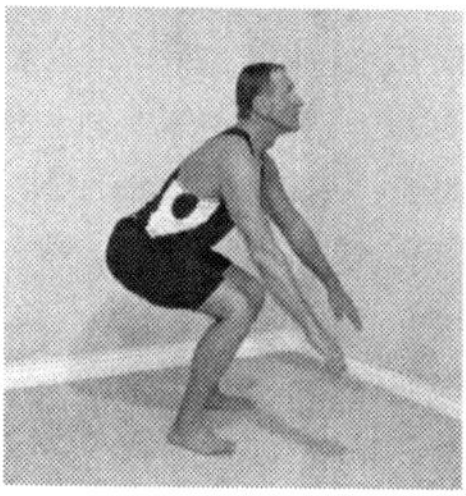

Figure #1

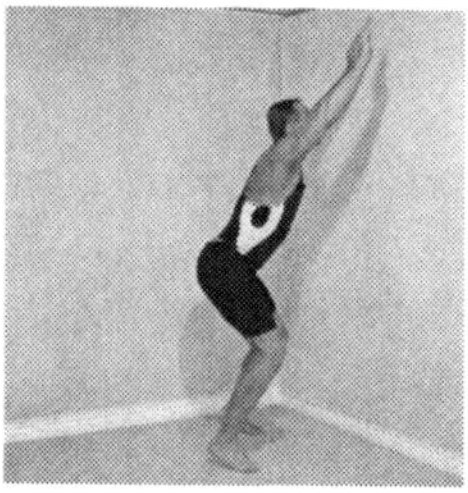

Figure #2

#90 – Box Jump

TARGET MUSCLE(S): Glutes, Quads, Calves, Hamstrings, Hip Flexors, Adductors

PROCEDURE: This exercise is similar to the Jump Squat. The difference is that you jump about 30 cm (12 inches) high to each of four corners (forward – sideways – backward – sideways). All four corners equal one rep. Start with 3-5 reps.

If it is helpful, you could have four small objects, placed appropriately in the shape of a square about 250-500mm apart (1-2 feet), to jump over. You may also want to start with a lower height and increase it over time.

#91 – Front to Back Jump Lunge

TARGET MUSCLE(S): Quads, Glutes, Hamstrings, Adductors, Hip Flexors, Calves

PROCEDURE: Start in a lunge position (Figure #1) and jump up while switching "forward" legs and moving back in to a lunge position (Figure #2). Try to hold the position for approximately 1-2 seconds before jumping each time so that you can intensify the load on your legs. This exercise will also help you practice your balance. Note that you always face forward for this exercise and maintain proper lunge form. You can keep your hands on your hips or at your sides as long as they are not on your legs.

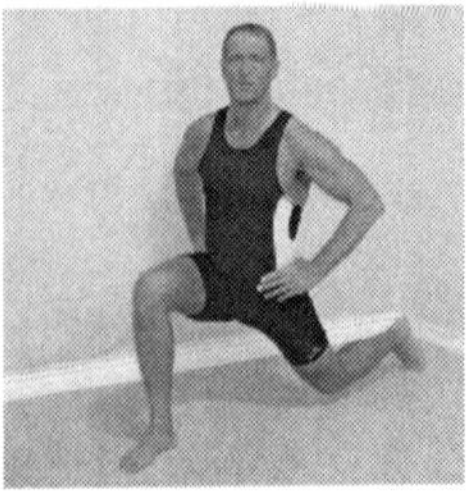

Figure #1 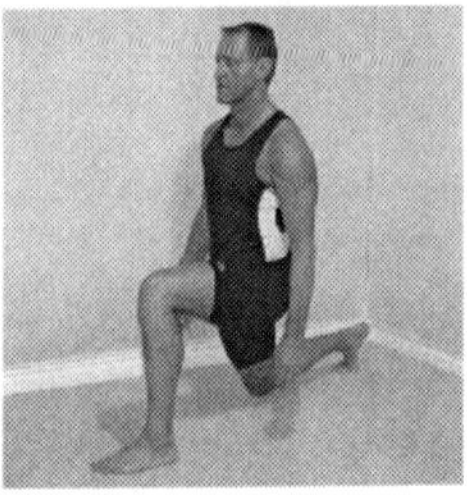   Figure #2

#92 – Jump Lunge – Directional Shift

TARGET MUSCLE(S): Glutes, Quads, Hamstrings, Calves, Hip Flexors, Adductors

PROCEDURE: This is a small variation of the Jump Lunge. The procedure is the same except when you jump up you change direction by 180 degrees (see below). When you move into the lunge position, you complete 1-5 lunges on that side before reversing and repeating the sequence on the other side. Complete lunges on both sides to equal one rep.

Remember to maintain proper form as it is easy to break during this exercise.

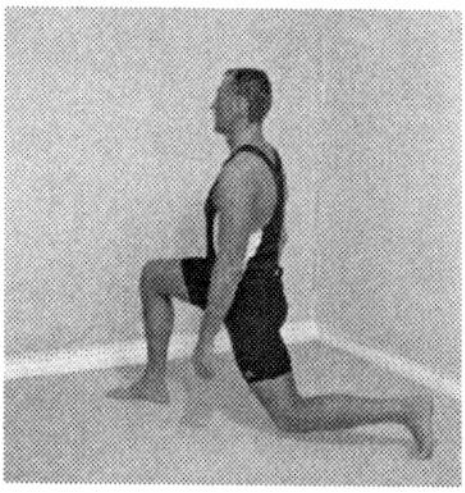

Figure #1

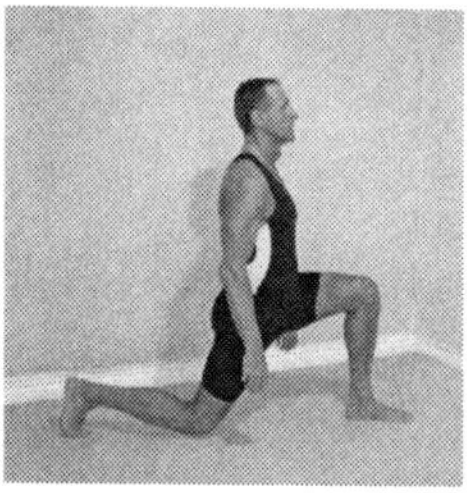

Figure #2

#93 – Mountain Climb

TARGET MUSCLE(S): Quads, Glutes, Calves, Hip Flexors, Delts, Triceps, Biceps, Abs

PROCEDURE: This drill is similar to the Leg Drive Push Up covered in the section on Resistance Training for the Upper Body. Maintain the Standard Push Up position (arms slightly bent) and alternately raise your knees into your chest utilizing a fast jump action (Figure #1). Remember to keep your back straight and your abs tight for the duration of the drill. Start with 5-10 reps on each leg.

A more intense variation of the Mountain Climb involves the same jump action but you raise your knees so they touch your elbows as shown in Figure #2. This will work the adductors and hip flexors and puts even more load on your deltoids. Ensure your knee touches your elbow, not lower. For a greater challenge and develop coordination, you could combine both variations by alternating each movement.

Figure #1   Figure #2

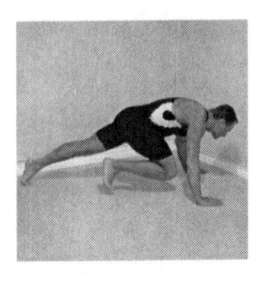

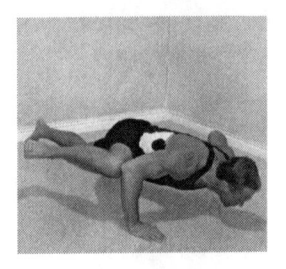

#94 – One Legged Jump

TARGET MUSCLE(S): Quads, Glutes, Hamstrings, Calves, Hip Flexors, Abs

PROCEDURE: This is a fairly straightforward exercise that involves standing erect, on one leg and on your toes, as shown below. While keeping your abs tight, jump up by pushing off from the leg you are standing on, and come down softly on the balls of your other foot. As soon as you land on your toes you should spring up instantly from that leg and land on the other. Effectively this becomes a "bouncing" motion. Start with 5-10 reps for each leg. If you find that one of your legs is stronger than the other, you could perform additional reps on the weaker leg to build up its strength.

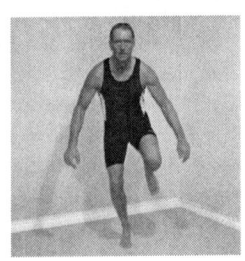

#95 – Belly Bashers (Advanced)

TARGET MUSCLE(S): Abs, Delts, Triceps, Biceps, Glutes, Quads, Hamstrings, Calves

PROCEDURE: This exercise definitely needs to be performed outdoors on a grassy surface. Even though all exercises in this section should be performed on a soft or outdoor grassy surface, it is particularly important for this one. Since it is more intense, try it only after attaining a high level of fitness.

It begins with running on the spot for about 5-10 seconds. You drop to the surface, in a push up position, but let your belly hit first as shown below (obviously your abs need to be flexed/tight at all times). Upon hitting the surface, immediately jump up and assume the spot running position. If you are uncomfortable with this approach to start with, you can drop into a push up position, without your abs hitting first, by cushioning the impact with your arms. You should start with only 3-5 reps as this is a fairly intense exercise.

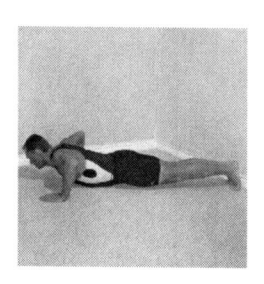

#96 – Step Ups

TARGET MUSCLE(S): Quads, Glutes, Calves, Hamstrings, Hip Flexors, Adductors

PROCEDURE: This exercise requires a stable/sturdy chair (a workout bench is ideal, if available). Stand in front of the chair (or at the side of your bench), approximately 75-100mm (3-4 inches) away, in the erect position. Step up on the chair and place your foot flat on it (Figure #1) while bringing up your other leg and just touching the chair with your toes without resting on it (Figure #2). While maintaining the erect position (do not hunch over), step down from the chair first with the leg that just touched the chair and follow with the other to return both legs to the surface. This sequence would represent one rep. Focus on the one side for the reps selected before switching to the other leg that would need to be flat on the chair. Try to keep your knee over the heel of the "chair" leg. Also try to keep your hands off your legs and at your side. A variation of this exercise involves performing shoulder circles (arms extended shoulder height) while stepping. Perform 5-10 reps each leg to start.

Figure #1

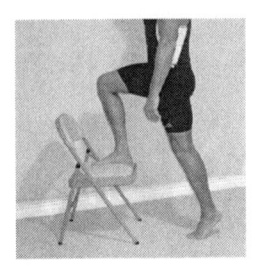

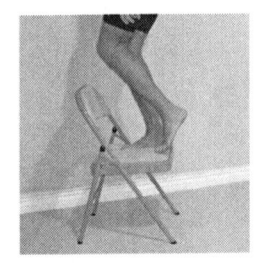

Figure #2

#97 – Burpee's (Advanced)

TARGET MUSCLE(S): Delts, Pecs, Triceps, Biceps, Abs, Hamstrings, Glutes, Quads, Calves

PROCEDURE: Start in a proper form Standard Squat position with your arms at your side (Figure #1). Leap as high as possible with your arms fully extended above your shoulders (Figure #2). When you return to the surface, immediately go in to a proper squat position for just a split second (Figure #1) and then extend your legs back to move into a Standard Push Up position (Figure #3). Complete a pushup (or any number you chose) and quickly leap back to the squat position as shown in Figure #1. Hold the squat position for a second before commencing the next rep. If you would like a further challenge, the number of and/or type of pushup(s) performed could be varied. Start with 5-10 reps.

NOTE: While you are in the process of learning this exercise, pause for a second between each step to check your form. There is a tendency to break proper squat form when you return from your jump and prior to performing the pushup.

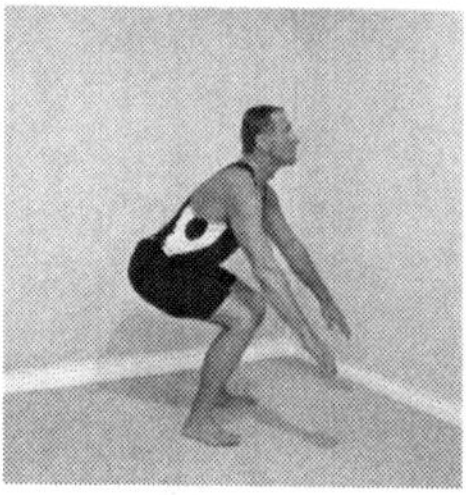

Figure #1

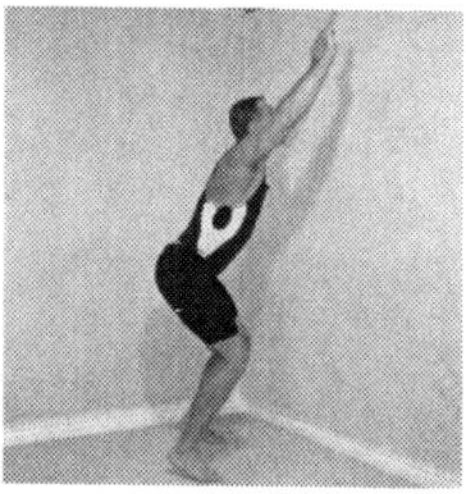

Figure #2

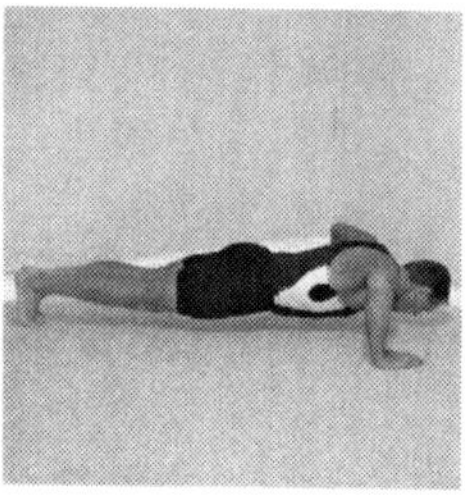

Figure #3

#98 – Karaoke

TARGET MUSCLE(S): Hip Flexors, Adductors, Calves, Glutes, Quads

PROCEDURE: Do this drill outdoors or in a place where there is room to run for at least 30-50 meters (or yards). Essentially this drill involves keeping your entire body facing forward while running sideways.

While running sideways cross your right leg over your left (Figure #1), then move your left leg sideways and finally cross your right leg behind the left as shown in Figure #2. Repeat this procedure for the distance and/or time you select. Once you have completed the distance/time selected, turn around 180 degrees and perform the same drill in the opposite direction. Cross your left leg over your right leg, then move your right leg sideways and finally cross your left leg behind your right leg.

Start with 50 yards or 20 seconds in duration and add distance/time/sets with improved fitness level.

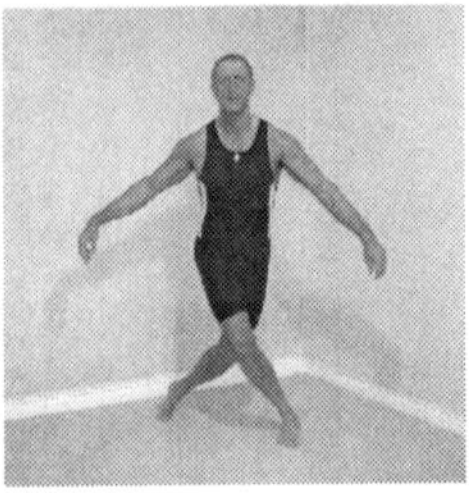

Figure #1

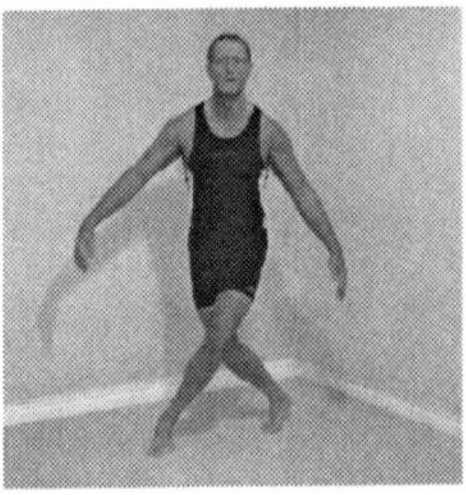

Figure #2

#99 – Kirtzie Karaoke (Advanced)

TARGET MUSCLE(S): Hamstrings, Glutes, Hip Flexors, Quads, Calves

PROCEDURE: This is a variation of the Karaoke drill. This is not only a good exercise for the target muscle group but it is also a good cardio drill. The key distinction is that it involves placing your palm on the surface between your legs when they are spread apart. Try walking through it first before you apply speed.

Begin with taking a lateral step, crossing your right leg over your left (Figure #1). Each time you cross your legs try to maintain a ½ metre (two foot) spread between them (you may need to work up to this) while you place your palm **flat** on the surface in front of you and between your legs (Figure #2). A "flat palm" enhances the load on the glutes due to the additional reach. Come up from placing your palm on the surface and reverse direction without stopping. Take two steps so you can cross your left leg over your right to complete a full rep.

Complete 5-10 reps in each direction to start. When you are comfortable with the exercise try increasing your speed and adding a small skip when changing direction.

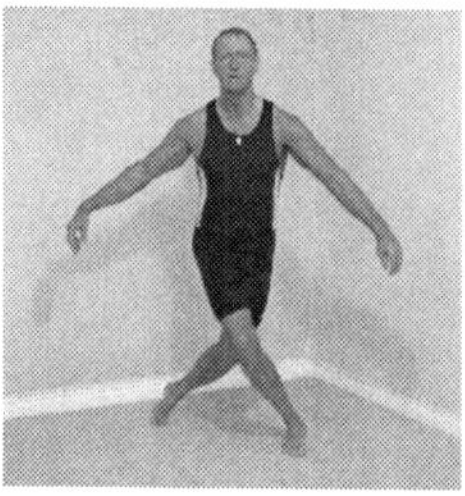

Figure #1

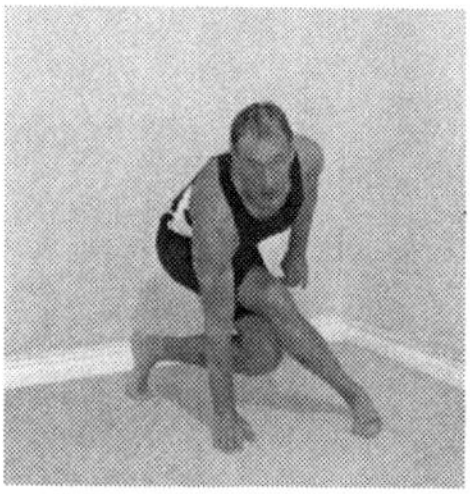

Figure #2

5. MARTIAL ARTS FOR STRENGTH & CARDIO

The exercises in this section are based on martial arts training. They have NOT been included to try and teach you martial arts and self defense as I firmly believe that these skills require a more "hands on" approach. They have been included because I have found from experience they can be a tremendous asset in terms of enhancing general physical fitness and also assist with the development of reflexes, coordination, speed, agility and quickness. I do not believe it matters what sport you play, hockey, baseball, soccer, football, or racquet sports, there are benefits that can be derived from martial arts and applied to your particular area of interest.

If you are not really interested in developing your speed or agility, for example, these exercises can still help improve overall physical fitness, especially your overall endurance and cardiovascular capacity. Furthermore, when executed properly they are a wonderful way to enhance muscle tone, and develop your abs and waist, while promoting leanness.

To gain the full benefit of the upcoming exercises and drills, it is essential that you understand the fundamentals of each martial arts form covered. Then you can use them effectively, ensuring that you always apply maximum effort. Keep in mind that you will find it much easier to maximize your effort throughout the drills if your abs remain firm during execution. This will also allow you to reach greater levels of intensity that will provide you an excellent "caloric burn" and cardio challenge.

It is important to understand that martial arts fundamentals require practice before they can be correctly executed. However, the return they provide, in terms of fitness, is well worth the effort. It takes many years of dedication and hard work for an individual to acquire a black belt in martial arts. I would never suggest that my years of training and teaching martial arts can easily be transferred to you in a few sessions with only a book as your guide. However, I can give you a basic understanding of the forms used in the drills covered in this section so that you can effectively execute them to enhance your physical fitness.

The following are some of the martial arts fundamentals that you need to understand:

1. Casual (training) Stance
2. Horse (training) Stance
3. Footwork
4. Punch
5. Kick
6. Block

Although I noted in an earlier chapter that your effort, time and commitment are essential for any successful fitness program, it is worth reinforcing "effort" here. Unless you apply maximum effort to each of the drills that use these fundamentals, you will not enjoy them as much or realize the physical fitness potential that is available.

A. FUNDAMENTALS

CASUAL (TRAINING) STANCE

This stance is a casual and comfortable position. Face forward with your shoulders square to your body. Keep your hands/fists level with your face, just below your eyes (proper fist form will be covered in the Punch). The positioning of the arms/hands will help assist with balance and also prepare you for other exercises and drills that utilize the kick, block and/or punch combinations.

Both of your legs should be bent slightly at your knees with one leg forward and the other slightly back (the toe of your back foot is even with the heel of your front foot). See Figure #1. With a focus on your front leg, turn your knee and your foot inward (Figure #2). Notice that the foot of your forward leg is flat on the surface to handle your body weight and provide balance. There is very little weight, if any, on the back foot and your heel does not touch the surface (Figure #2). This stance will be covered further when the Kick and Footwork are reviewed.

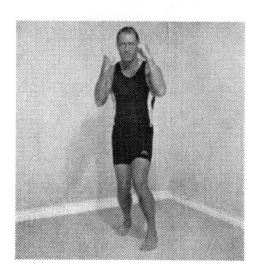

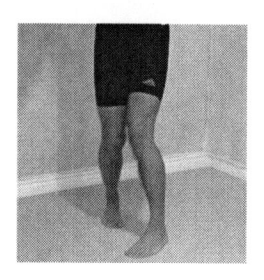

Figure #1   Figure #2

HORSE (TRAINING) STANCE

This effective training stance is similar to sitting in a saddle when riding a horse (hence the name). Your legs are straddled, as shown below, while you try to squat down to a level where your quads and hamstrings are level with the surface (or as close as you can get). Also note that your knees should be over your heels and your toes pointed forward (heels pushed out). Your upper body should be erect and your shoulders square. Ideally, the weight of your body is shifted forward, or on the balls of your feet.

If you are in a proper "Horse Stance", typically you will notice tension on your adductors and perhaps your glutes almost right away. You should try to maintain this isometric position for the duration of punch or block drills.

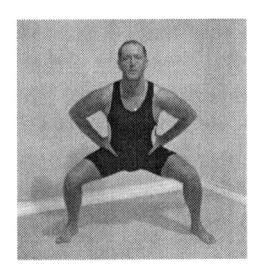

PUNCH

It may seem that executing a punch is quite straightforward, however, there are key aspects that you need to understand so that you can make your workout more effective and avoid potential injury.

The first thing you need to know is how to make a proper fist so you can avoid potential hyperextension of your elbow. Quite simply, all you do is tuck your thumb behind your fingers, when you make a fist, as shown in Figure #1. Your fist must be tight when performing any punch or block drill.

Your abs should ALWAYS be tight when executing a punch (even a block). This increases the effectiveness of the drill.

When executing a punch, extend your arm approximately chest level but maintain a very slight bend at your elbow (Figure #2). This will help avoid potential hyperextension of the elbow. While you execute the punch with one arm, pull your opposite arm back to your side (Figure #3). Notice that the knuckles of the fist pulled back are facing down while the knuckles of the "punching fist" are facing up – **this is important**. This transition of the knuckles actually occurs in the last few inches (75 mm) of the punch as it is executed. Also notice how the hip shifts as the punch is delivered as shown in Figure #2. This is where your power comes from while enhancing caloric burn. A right punch is delivered with the right hip while the left leg bends slightly outward. A left punch would involve the opposite. I suggest that you practice this technique in slow motion, or in front of a mirror to gain comfort, before using it in a drill.

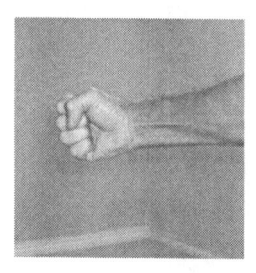

Figure #1

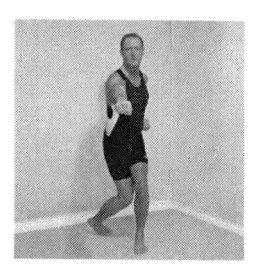

Figure #2

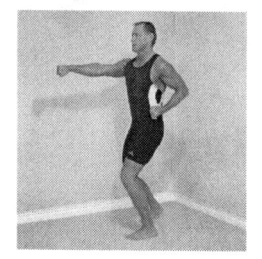

Figure #3

KICK

For a kick to be effective and useful for training purposes there are some basics you need to know. Start with the Casual Stance as covered previously. Both legs should be bent slightly for maneuverability (Figure #1). When executing a kick, always curl your toes back as shown in Figure #2. This will help prevent potential hyperextension of your knee.

The kick actually involves four steps. However, when executed with speed it looks like one. First, lift your knee to your hip from the Casual Stance position – this is a quick action (Figure #3); then, snap your foot forward from your knee (Figure #4) so it is level with your hip and quickly return it (Figure #3); and finally return your "kicking leg" to its original position (Figure #1).

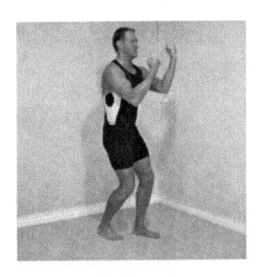

Figure #1

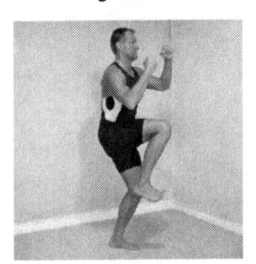

Figure #2

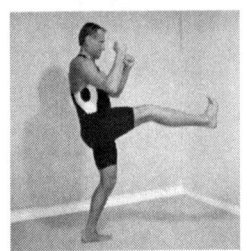

Figure #3

Figure #4

BLOCK

The block draws from some of the aspects used in the punch. Your abs remain tight while the movement of your hip, hands and arms are similar.

In a casual training stance, raise your arm to your side so that your elbow is approximately shoulder level and bent 90 degrees as shown in Figure #1. Notice that your fist is positioned so that your knuckles are pointed towards you. When you execute a block, you bring your bent upper arm across the front of your body, approximately chest level, and turn your fist so that your knuckles are facing away from you. Shift your hips slightly (left hip with a left block and vice versa) while you perform the block (Figure #2).

As you execute the block, pull your opposite arm back (with a tight fist) to your side as also shown in Figure #2. Your knuckles face down consistent with the punch. I suggest that also you practice this technique in slow motion, or in front of a mirror, before using it in a drill.

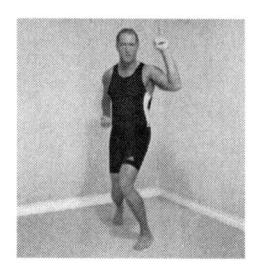

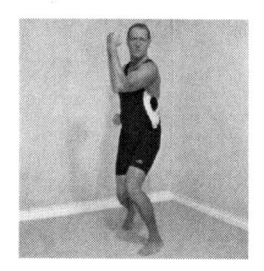

Figure #1   Figure #2

FOOTWORK

To assist with proper kick, block, punch and line drills, it is essential to maintain proper footwork. Developing your footwork can also assist with improving your co-ordination, speed and agility. Developing good footwork places demands on your hips and, since the hips are the largest bone structure in your body, they provide you with the greatest leverage and force. This leverage from the hips ultimately transfers speed down through your legs to your feet.

You can start to work on your footwork using the Casual Stance covered earlier (Figure #1). Practice by moving around in different directions and switching your forward foot periodically. Always watch your feet, legs and hips while you are preparing to deliver a punch (a mirror can be very helpful). In the Casual Stance position, you can also practice lifting your back foot off the surface, to check your balance periodically, prior to delivering a Kick.

With your weight shifted to your front foot it will be easier to maneuver and utilize your back foot for a Kick (Figure #2), or a Punch (Figure #3) or to move your body sideways for a Punch drill (Figure #4). Remember that you always pivot/move on the balls of your feet.

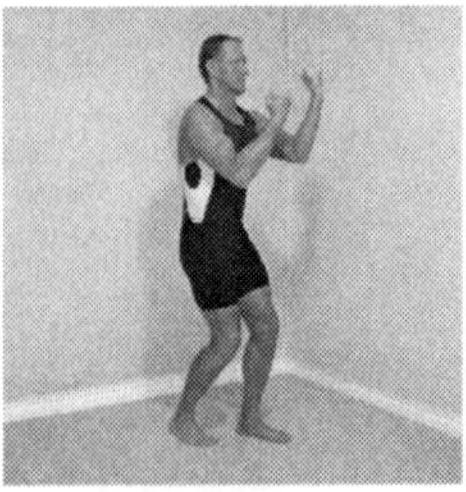

Figure #1

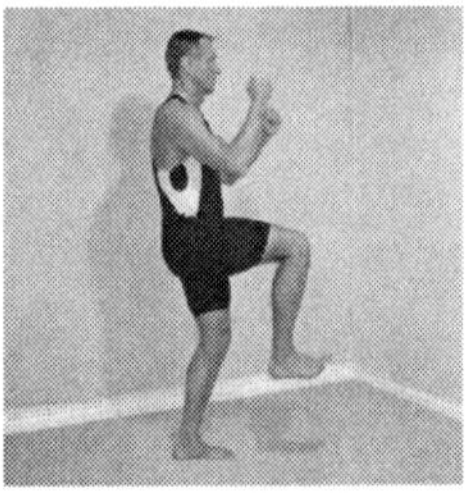

Figure #2

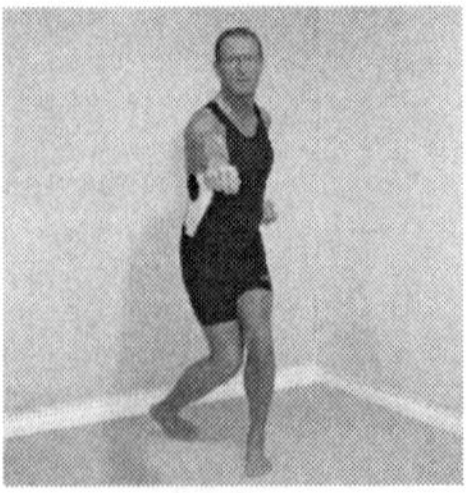

Figure #3

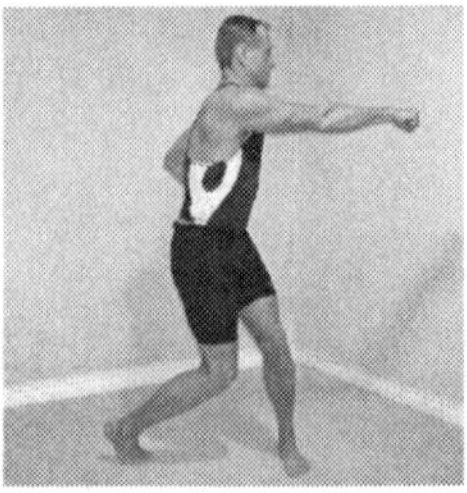

Figure #4

B. APPLYING THE FUNDAMENTALS

You can utilize the techniques we have just covered to develop great drills to challenge your body in terms of muscular and cardiovascular development. They are especially beneficial when they are combined with the numerous exercises and suggested programs included in this guide. If you practice these fundamentals and perform them properly you will come to appreciate the level of enjoyment you can draw from them. You'll also be pleasantly surprised with the caloric burn they provide.

To ensure that you realize a good workout from the following martial arts based drills, please remember that it is essential for you to apply "your" maximum effort. As your fitness level improves you can increase sets and reps just as you would for any other type of exercise included in this guide. A good starting point for any of the drills that follow would be one set of 5-10 reps.

Although previously stated, it is worth reinforcing that you will need to be mindful of your form. Proper form is crucial, especially with martial arts techniques, as it will maximize the benefits you receive in terms of enhanced physical fitness while reducing the risk of potential injury to tendons, joints and muscles.

#100 - Punch Drill – Casual Stance

TARGET MUSCLE(S): Abs, Obliques, Biceps, Triceps, Delts, Pecs

PROCEDURE: Execute a right punch directed at a 45 degree angle from the direction you are facing as shown in Figure #1. To perform a left punch you simply switch your foot placement and follow the same procedure (Figure #3). Notice the placement of the hands/arms while transitioning from the right punch to completing the left punch as shown in Figure #2.

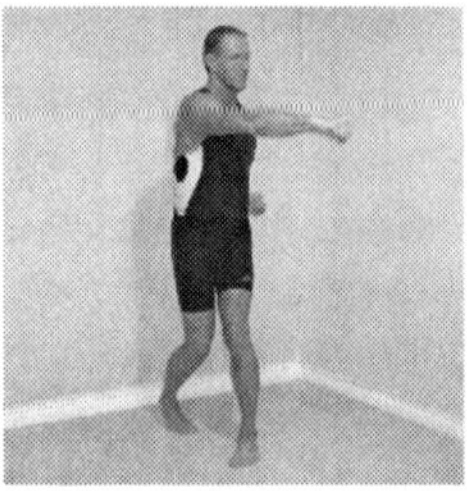

Figure #1

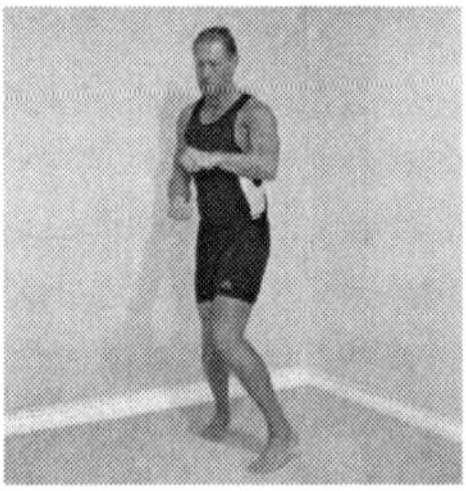

Figure #2

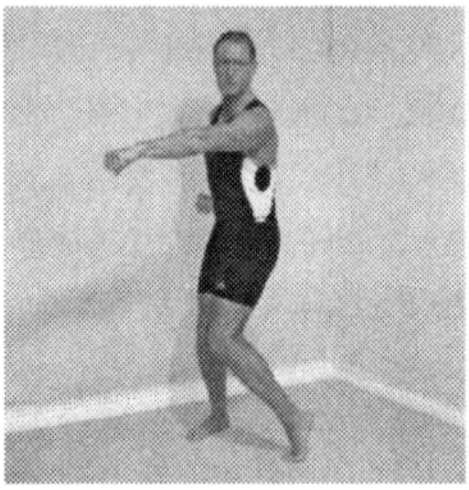

Figure #3

As you become more comfortable with this drill you can execute the right and left punches in succession without stopping. This will significantly enhance your workout. Remember to pivot on both feet, while changing direction, so you can easily transfer your weight from one foot to the other. As you change your direction, your punch follows. Your back foot always determines what punch you are throwing (right foot back – right punch; left foot back – left punch). This allows you to use your hip to lever your punch.

For the purposes of your workout, a left and right punch is one rep.

#101 - Punch Drill – Horse Stance

TARGET MUSCLE(S): Glutes, Quads, Hamstrings, Adductors, Abs, Obliques, Biceps, Triceps

PROCEDURE: When you execute a punch in this stance it is more straightforward. In the Horse Stance shown below (Figure #1) throw a punch with either arm while pulling back with the other and placing it at your side (Figure #2). Apply the same steps to the other side to complete 1 rep. Ensure you hold the deep Horse Stance position to effectively work the adductors and hip flexors (they will burn if this drill is executed correctly).

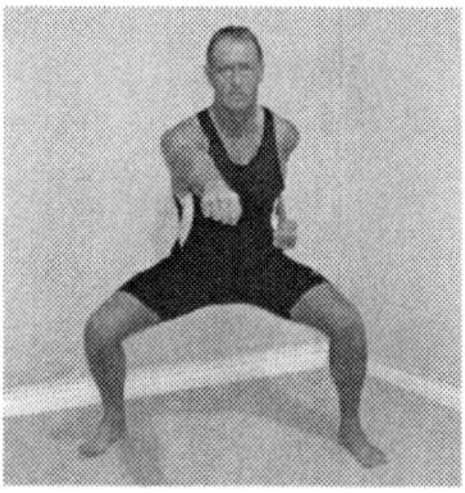

Figure #1 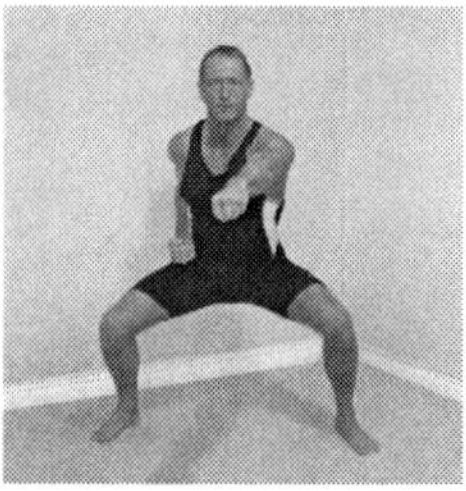   Figure #2

#102 - Upper Cut Drill

TARGET MUSCLE(S): Glutes, Quads, Hamstrings, Adductors Abs, Obliques, Delts, Pecs, Triceps, Biceps

PROCEDURE: Assume the Casual Stance position. Crouch down slightly and move to a 45 degree angle by shifting your hips and feet. Make sure you keep your back relatively straight (Figure #1). This will prepare you for unloading the punch. Rise up as you execute the punch as shown in Figure #2 (notice this is a short punch that does not involve fully extending your arm), and crouch down as you shift direction, but maintain your Casual Stance. It's somewhat like a "bob and weave" motion.

As you shift from side to side you will also change your front foot. When you move left as shown in Figure #3 you lead with your left leg and punch with your right fist. When you shift to the right as shown in Figure #1, you lead with your right leg while you punch with your left fist.

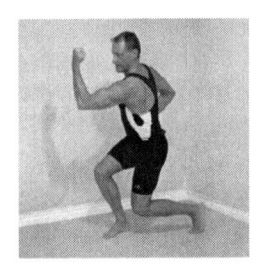

Figure #1

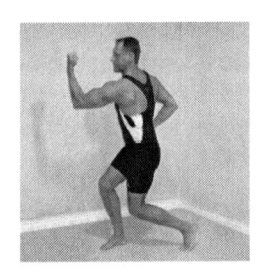

Figure #2

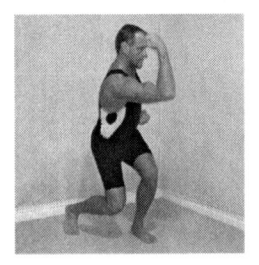

Figure #3

#103 - Power Punch Drill

TARGET MUSCLE(S): Abs, Obliques, Delts, Pecs, Triceps, Biceps

PROCEDURE: In the Casual Stance move 180 degrees from the direction you are facing while shifting your hips and feet. While you turn to the side, execute a standard punch, approximately chest level, and do not straighten your arm completely (Figure #1). Shift to the opposite direction and repeat the procedure (Figure #3). Take note of the positioning of the hands and arms, while transitioning from one side to the other, to set up execution of the next punch (Figure #2).

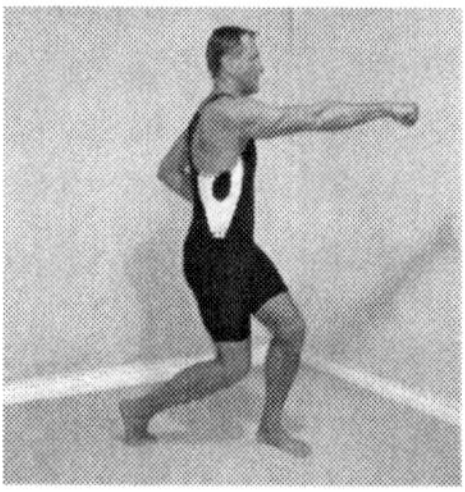

Figure #1

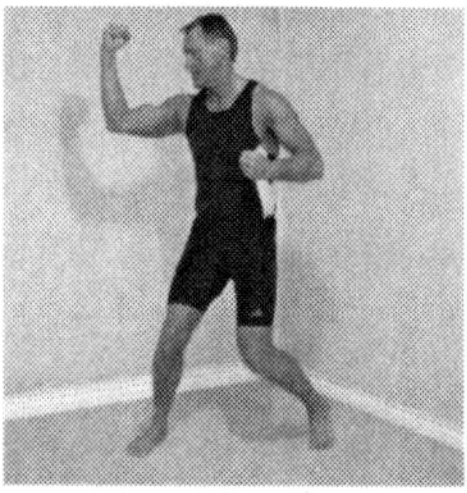

Figure #2

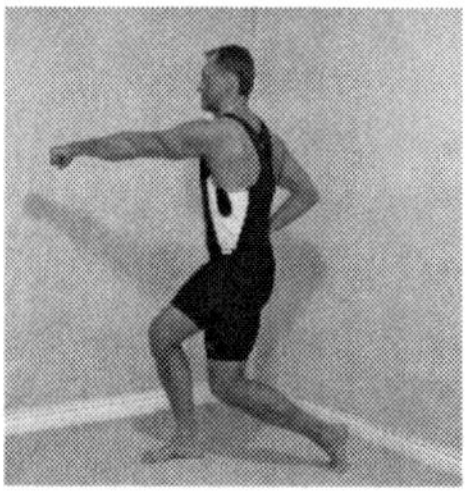

Figure #3

The Power Punch can also be executed while in the Horse Stance. Essentially, the same technique is followed as described above except the punch is straight ahead. An even further challenge would involve punching (reaching) about a 135 degree angle. There is no hip and foot movement in the Horse Stance when executing a punch. However, this approach works the shoulders, lats and abs in terms of the upper body and also the adductors while maintaining the Horse Stance.

#104 - Rabbit Punch Drill

TARGET MUSCLE(S): Abs, Obliques, Delts, Pecs, Triceps, Biceps

PROCEDURE: This drill is essentially the same as the Power Punch drill. You begin with the Casual or Horse Stance and perform the same type of punch. The difference is that you complete three, or more, hard rapid and consecutive punches before reversing direction and repeating. Speed is essential for this drill to be effective. Another option is to apply multiple upper cut punches one direction and then shift.

#105 - Elbow Punch Drill

TARGET MUSCLE(S): Abs, Obliques, Delts, Triceps

PROCEDURE: The Elbow Punch is similar to the Power Punch in terms of form and movement. The only difference is that you execute a punch with your elbow instead of your fist. This is done by quickly raising your elbow as high as your head with your fist drawn into your chest. Shift your hips, like a typical punch, while thrusting the elbow up and forward (see below). Repeat the technique, shifting to the other side, as you would with the Power Punch.

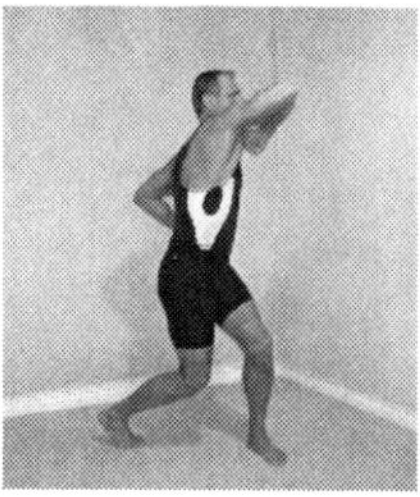

#106 - Combination Punch Drill

TARGET MUSCLE(S): Abs, Obliques, Delts, Pecs, Triceps, Biceps

PROCEDURE: This drill combines multiple punch techniques covered previously. One option could involve the execution of a Power Punch in one direction (Figure #1) and quickly shifting the opposite direction to perform an Upper Cut Punch (Figure #2). Once you have completed the drill following your selected format you would need to switch direction/sides and repeat. When changing direction, always remember to step through while shifting your hips and feet.

As you gain comfort with the different types of punches, change the punches you use in combination to mix up the drills. Incorporate the Upper Cut Punch, Power Punch, Rabbit Punch, and Rapid Fire Punch, on a regular basis so your body is continually challenged. I recommend you gain comfort with the form of the different types of punches before combining them.

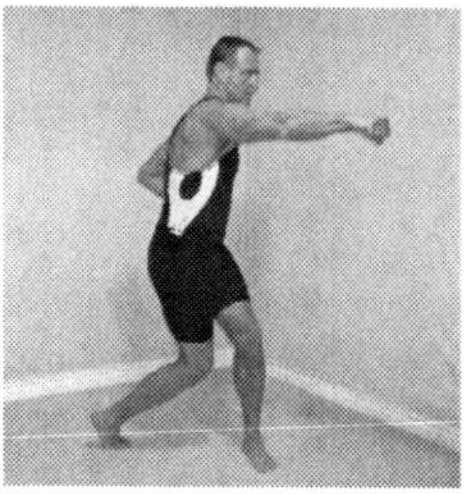

Figure #1 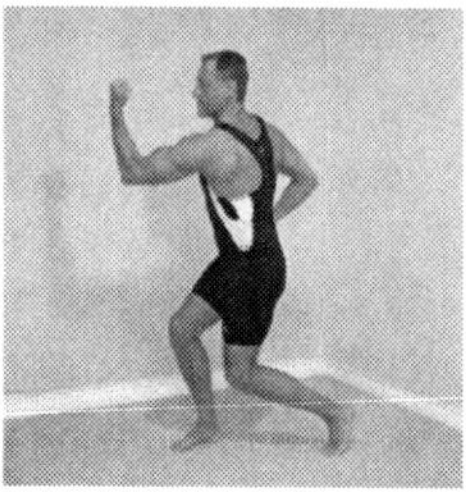   Figure #2

#107 - Front Kick Drill

TARGET MUSCLE(S): Hamstrings, Glutes, Quads, Hip Flexors, Adductors, Calves, Abs

PROCEDURE: One option for this drill involves executing multiple kicks (reps) with one leg before switching to the other. Ensure you move back to the traditional training stance for a split second in between each kick executed (Figure #1). Essentially this would mean simply touching your kicking toe to the surface to maintain balance before quickly performing the next kick. This also provides another way to enhance your drill and workout. Another option is to alternate legs with each kick you execute (a good caloric burn).

Please note the positioning of the arms/hands, while kicking, in Figure #2. This will help assist with balance and also prepare you for other drills that utilize kick/punch combinations.

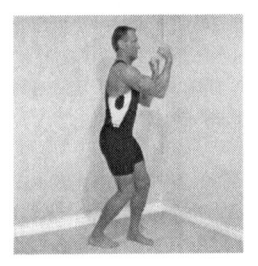

Figure #1

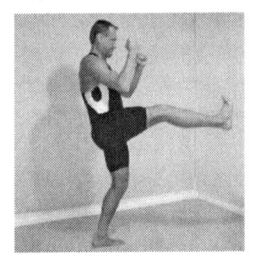

Figure #2

#108 - Side Kick Drill

TARGET MUSCLE(S): Hamstrings, Glutes, Quads, Hip Flexors, Adductors, Calves, Abs, Obliques

PROCEDURE: Follow the technique described for a Front Kick with the Casual Stance (Figure #1). Bend to your side as far as possible (90 degrees is ideal) before kicking 90

degress to the side of your body and waist high (Figure #2). Return to the Casual Stance between each kick executed.

Try to make sure that you shift your hips when performing the kick and that your forward foot has also shifted so that the heel of that foot faces the direction you are kicking (Figure #2). This will also assist with your balance. Focus on kicking with one leg before shifting over to the other side. When you gain comfort, another more challenging approach involves alternating kicks with each leg (another good caloric burn).

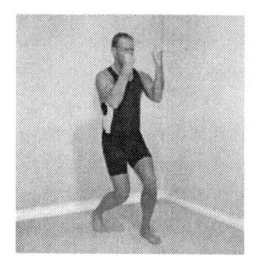

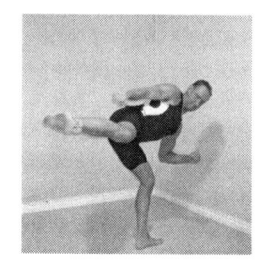

Figure #1

Figure #2

#109 - Rabbit Kick Drill

TARGET MUSCLE(S): Hamstrings, Glutes, Quads, Hip Flexors, Adductors, Calves, Abs

PROCEDURE: This drill also uses the Front Kick. The minor, yet challenging, difference is that the kicks (reps) you execute are all done in succession. This involves executing the kicks by rapidly snapping them from your knee without returning to the Casual Stance until you are done. This drill can also use the Side Kick and the Rear Kick by holding their respective positions. This is also a very good drill for practicing your balance.

#110 - Rear Kick Drill

TARGET MUSCLE(S): Hamstrings, Glutes, Quads, Hip Flexors, Adductors, Calves, Abs

PROCEDURE: From the Casual Stance position (Figure #1) lean over at a 90 degree angle. As you bend over, bring your knee into your chest as close as possible (Figure #2). As soon as you have drawn your knee in, quickly extend your leg so that it is parallel with the surface (make sure you push through your heel - Figure #3). Immediately thereafter, bring your knee back into your chest (Figure #2) before lowering it to the surface and returning to the Casual Stance (Figure #1). Focus on one side before changing.

To intensify this drill, you can maintain the bent over position while performing successive kicks similar to the Rabbit Kick described previously. This is most effective for the glutes while enhancing your caloric burn. Another option involves alternating legs with each kick.

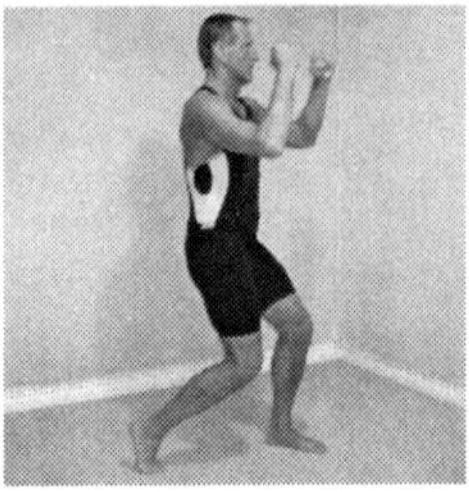

Figure #1

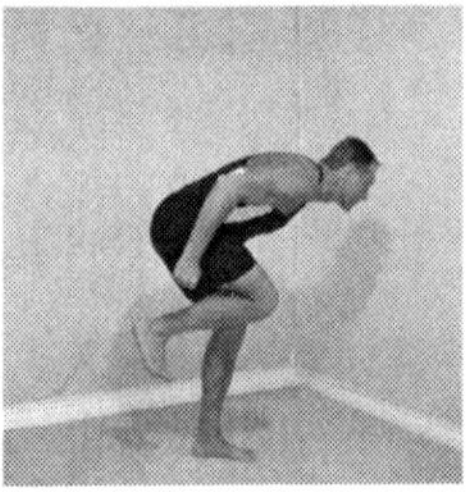

Figure #2

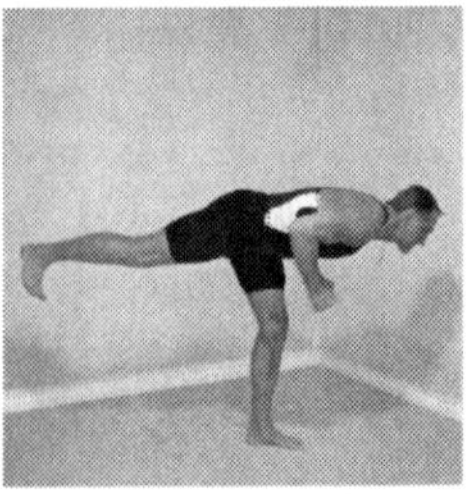

Figure #3

#111 - Crab Kick Drill

TARGET MUSCLE(S): Hamstrings, Glutes, Quads, Hip Flexors, Adductors, Calves, Abs, Obliques

PROCEDURE: Sit down and rest on your elbows (just as if you are sitting on the floor watching television). Bring one of your legs in towards you so your knee is at a 90 degree angle to your hips while you execute a kick shown in Figure #1. Once you are comfortable with this drill, you could increase the intensity by raising your body so that it maintains a level position with the surface. From this position, you perform a front alternating kick (Figure #2). Keep your abs tight and do not drop your lower body.

As you gain comfort you can further enhance the drill by kicking sideways at a 45 degree angle. Ensure you cross over your bent leg when switching from side to side as shown in Figure #3.

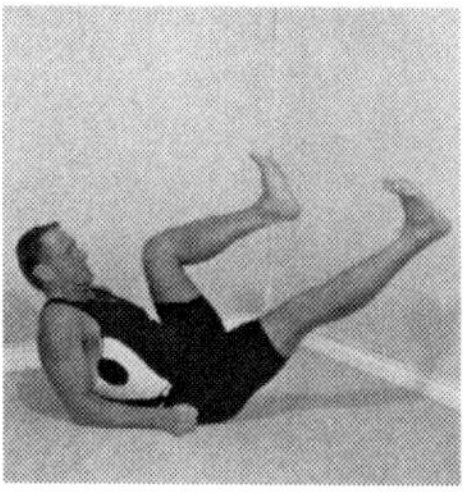

Figure #1

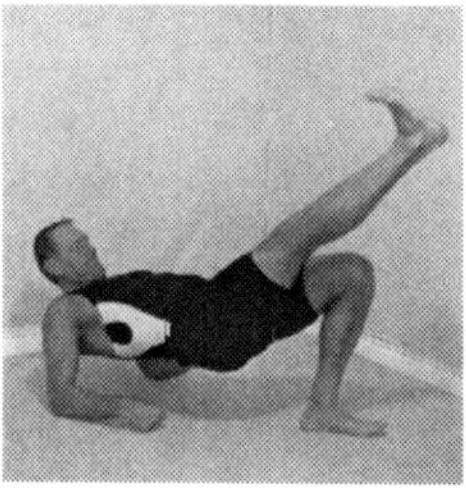

Figure #2

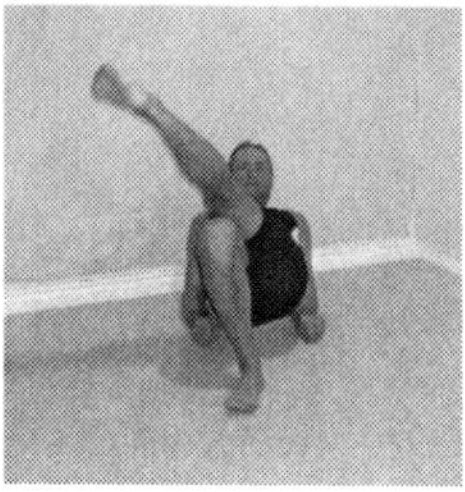

Figure #3

#112 - Front/Rear Kick Combination

TARGET MUSCLE(S): Hamstrings, Glutes, Quads, Hip Flexors, Adductors, Calves, Abs

PROCEDURE: This drill combines the Front and Rear Kicks (front then rear or vice versa) in succession (Figures #1 and #3 below).

To gain the greatest benefit from this drill, try to perform it as fast as possible while maintaining proper form. However, you will need to practice this before increasing your speed. Until you gain comfort with this drill, you might try touching your toes of the "kicking" foot on the surface to gain balance before moving to the next kick (Figure #2). Over time, the ideal form does not include touching the "kicking foot" to the surface when moving from the front to the rear kick. This not only helps with developing balance and co-ordination but is a wonderful caloric burn.

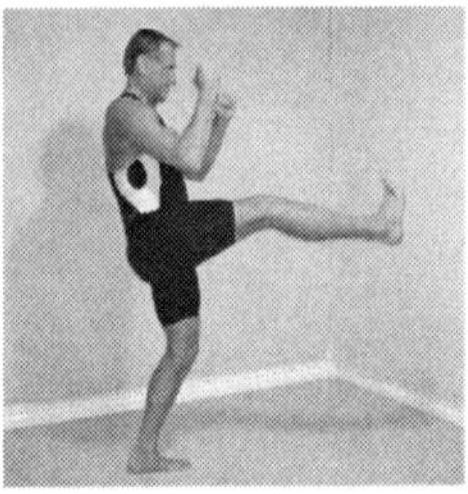

Figure #1

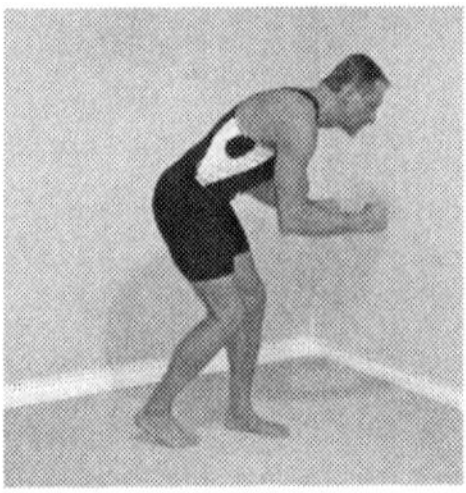

Figure #2

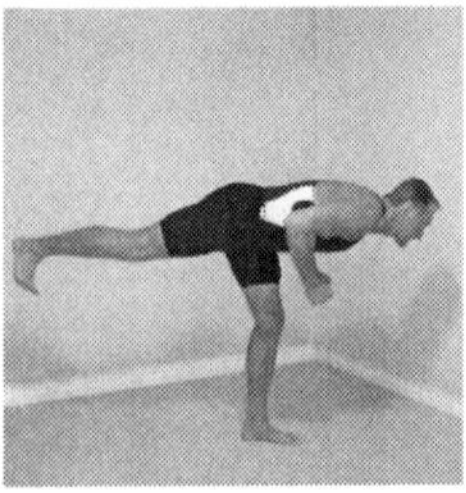

Figure #3

#113 - Front/Side/Rear Kick Combination

TARGET MUSCLE(S): Hamstrings, Glutes, Quads, Hip Flexors, Adductors, Calves, Abs, Obliques

PROCEDURE: This drill combines all three kicks previously covered. Start in the Casual Stance and execute a Front Kick (Figure #1); then perform a Side Kick (Figure #2) and finish with a Rear Kick (Figure #3). Although you can perform the three kicks in any order, I recommend you stay with the order suggested and return to the Casual Stance, for a split second between each kick, until you gain comfort with the drill. All three kicks should be executed in succession to complete 1 repetition.

A good test of endurance, agility, balance and coordination involves completing all kicks before placing the "kicking" foot on the surface. Another challenge involves following with an alternating set of kicks on the other side without a rest or pause between.

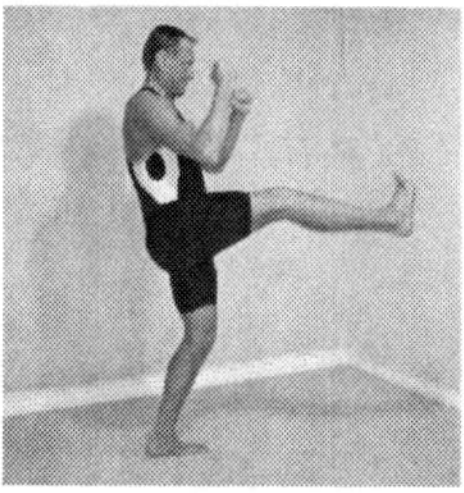

Figure #1

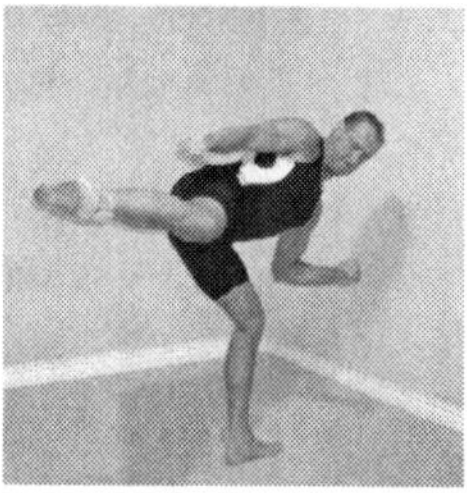

Figure #2

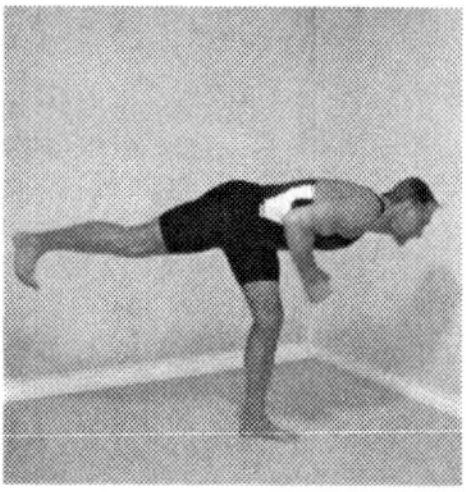

Figure #3

#114 - Block/Punch/Kick Combinations

TARGET MUSCLE(S): Hamstrings, Glutes, Quads, Hip Flexors, Adductors, Calves, Abs, Obliques, Triceps, Biceps, Pecs, Delts

PROCEDURE: This is an excellent drill that challenges a larger group of muscles. It will also test numerous areas of development including stamina, endurance, balance, coordination, speed and even strength. The drill is accomplished by combining any of the previously described punches, block and kicks together as one rep (yes, one rep without stopping).

When you perform this drill, always move from one side of your body to the other regardless of the combinations being executed. This helps to provide a balanced muscle workout. For example, you could execute a left Block (Figure #1); followed by a right Power Punch (Figure #2) and finish with a right Front Kick (Figure #3). Another example might be to execute a right Block, a left Upper Cut followed by a left Side Kick or left Front Kick, and so on. Always keep in mind that you want to continue to switch from side to side, with each technique and/or combination executed, so that you gain a balanced full body muscular workout.

Figure #1

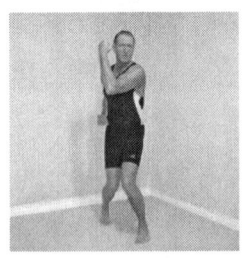

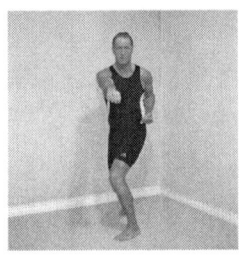

Figure #2

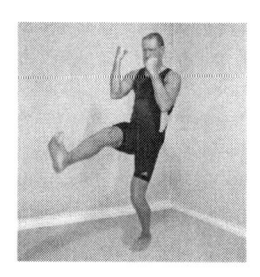

Figure #3

#115 - Shadow Sparring Drill

TARGET MUSCLE(S): All muscle groups previously noted

PROCEDURE: This is an effective anaerobic drill that involves all of the techniques and drills covered in this section. Quite simply, just pretend you are engaged in a competitive "match" with an imaginary opponent. You constantly move around in a small area while randomly executing punches, kicks and blocks. You will need to use maximum effort with each move so that you gain highest cardio and muscle toning benefit. Try to perform each "round" for about 10-15 seconds to start and rest for the same amount of time. This would constitute one set. Shadow Sparring provides a great caloric burn!

#116 – Line Drill

TARGET MUSCLE(S): All muscle groups previously noted

PROCEDURE: This is another effective anaerobic drill. It is similar to Shadow Sparring except you perform a series of specific moves, which you select, facing one direction and then mirror execution of the moves in the opposite direction.

You continue doing the "Line Drill" until you have finished the total number of reps or sets you want to complete.

As an example, you could execute a Power Punch, a Front Kick and an Upper Cut Punch in sequence facing one direction, without rest. Upon completion of the three moves, immediately throw another Power Punch, while you step through and move into the opposite direction, so that the punch is actually directed in the opposite direction you are moving. Follow with another Front Kick and Upper Cut Punch to complete the rep (the three moves that you execute in each direction count as one rep). The key to this drill is that there is no stopping for a rest when changing direction.

You can mix up the type and number of moves you select for the Line Drill. I suggest you practice a few sets at slow speed until you are comfortable with your combination. Thereafter, maximum effort and speed will deliver positive results in terms of speed, agility, quickness, coordination and caloric burn.

6. STRETCHING AND COOL DOWN

Generally speaking, as you age, the stretching component of a workout becomes even more important. It's been suggested that regular stretching can even help delay the aging process. In my opinion, the stretching aspect of a workout is essential as it sets the stage for further progress no matter what your goals may be. It should not be treated as an afterthought, or something you do quickly just to fit it in at the end of your workout. Most of your workout should have involved hard work so the end of your workout should be more relaxing, slow and gradual. Your body deserves this reward.

The stretching exercises included in this guide incorporate many related Yoga techniques to help provide a soothing and relaxing mind and body experience. A very light stretch just before going to bed can even help you sleep.

Stretching not only helps to maintain posture and flexibility but it also helps to prepare your body for the next workout by lengthening the muscles and creating a wider ROM. To appreciate the benefits from stretching I'd like you to think of your muscles in terms of a rubber band. If you try to stretch a rubber band too quickly, especially when it is cold, it could snap because it is tight. If the rubber band is warmed up, and you stretch it slowly and gradually, it will become longer, have more elasticity and be more responsive when you pull (stretch) it even further the next time. This is why maintaining your flexibility will help you avoid potential injury and make everyday activities much easier.

This is also why stretching assists with muscular and cardiovascular development in the longer term because it helps you get more out of your body, in terms of performance, when you need it.

The stretching component of a workout should normally take 10-30 minutes and be the last activity you complete. It helps prepare the body for its next workout, as already mentioned (improved muscle response), and it also complements a proper cool down. It does this by helping to gradually lower the heart rate and removing the lactic acid from your body that has built up from exercising.

The stretching movement should always be performed in a slow, gentle and relaxed manner. It should be challenging but not to the point of being painful. When releasing from a stretch, the motion should be gradual to avoid potential injury. To assist with the stretching experience and promote a more effective cool down, it is helpful to practice the breathing technique (pranayama) that was discussed in a previous section.

The types of stretching techniques shown in this chapter are stationary or "static". This means that you take one or more of your joints through a full range of motion, to an end point of slight discomfort, and hold it for a period of time. An after workout stretch can involve "static" stretching because the muscles and joints are warmed up (remember the rubber band analogy). This is even more important if the muscles are tight from a previous workout. In this case, performing these types of stretches before warming up could increase the risk of pulling a muscle or sustaining an injury.

Each stretch should be performed for **20-30 seconds minimum.** Ideally, the associated stretch for each joint should be performed 2-3 times (pause slightly for about 5 seconds between each set). I might add there are numerous opinions on this topic. The number and type of stretches completed after a workout typically depends on the areas of the body that were worked, for example upper body, lower body and/or cardio, abs and back. The stretching component of the workout is also impacted by the degree of intensity applied to the workout itself. A more demanding workout should incorporate a longer stretch period.

Although certainly not exhaustive, the stretching exercises included in this section are intended to provide you with a wide variety to choose from for your own program. You might vary the stretching exercises you use on a regular basis within your program. This way your body will continue to be challenged and not become comfortable or lazy due to its familiarity with the stretching exercises you utilize.

The stretches that follow are grouped in the same manner as the training exercises that have been provided:

   a. Lower Body
   b. Upper Body
   c. Abs, Back and Neck

The stretches that follow each address a number of muscles or muscle groups. However, the "Target Muscle(s)" of focus that are identified typically note only the primary muscle(s) or group and not all of the muscles that benefit from each stretch.

A. LOWER BODY

#117 - Leg Splits

TARGET MUSCLE(S): Hamstrings

PROCEDURE: Rest your back knee on the surface while maintaining an upright position. Extend your front leg with your toes pointed up (Figure #1). To enhance the stretch, you can place your palms flat on the surface on each side of your fully extended knee shown in Figure #2. Pivot to the other side and repeat the procedure.

As you become more comfortable with this stretch you can try extending your back leg as much as possible while maintaining your palms on the surface (Figure #3).

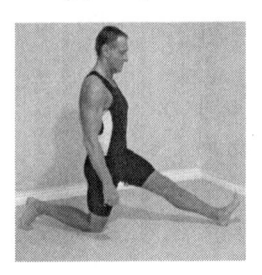

Figure #1

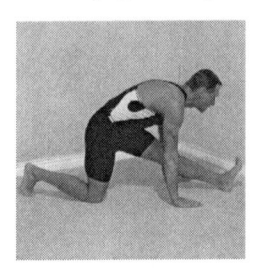

Figure #2

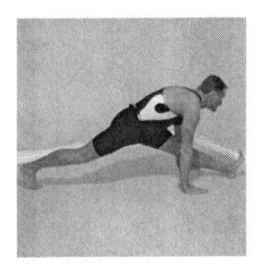

Figure #3

#118 - Single Vertical Leg

TARGET MUSCLE(S): Hamstrings

PROCEDURE: Lie on your back and place one leg flat on the surface while your other leg is vertically extended against the wall corner. It is important to ensure your knee remains flat against the wall as shown in Figure #1.

If you want to stretch your glutes, while in this position, simply cross your leg over your knee. You can enhance this part of the stretch by placing gentle pressure on your knee with your hand as shown in Figure #2. If a wall is not available, you could try holding onto your toes while keeping both legs fully extended as shown in Figure #3.

The key is to maintain fully extended legs so you may need to reach lower, perhaps to your knees, in order to do so. To increase the hamstring stretch, you could hold onto the toes of your keg that is vertically extended while your other leg is extended along the surface (Figure #4).

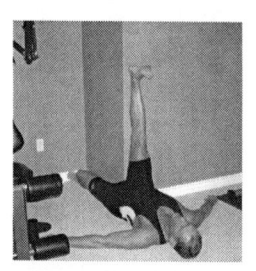

Figure #1

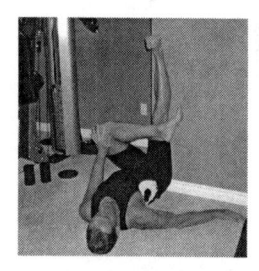

Figure #2

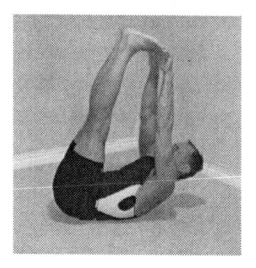

Figure #3

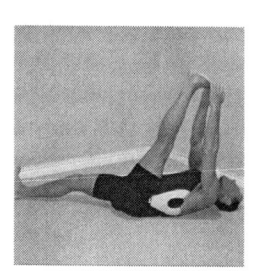

Figure #4

#119 - Leg Spread 1

TARGET MUSCLE(S): Adductors, Hamstrings

PROCEDURE: Lie on your back, bend your legs and hold onto your toes. Extend your legs laterally as wide as possible (Figure #1). If it is difficult to extend your legs while holding onto your toes, try holding the **inside** of your legs at your ankle or calf muscle (Figure #2). You can gradually work up to holding your toes. It is important to keep your legs fully extended to gain the best stretch for the adductors and hamstrings. For the final step, pull down on your legs to intensify the stretch.

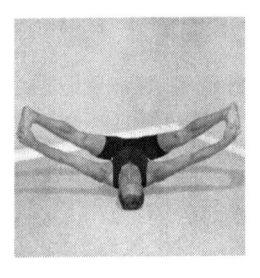

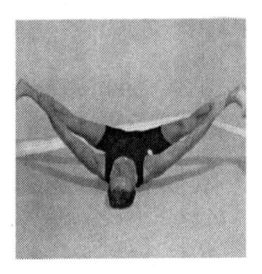

Figure #1   Figure #2

#120 - Leg Spread 2

TARGET MUSCLE(S): Adductors, Hamstrings

PROCEDURE: Bend over and spread your legs as wide as comfortably possible. Try to keep your feet pointed forward and draw an imaginary line between your toes. Cross your arms and try to place them on the line, as shown below. It may take some practice before being able to perform this stretch as pictured so you may need to work up to it by gradually lowering the arms each time.

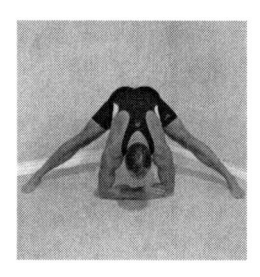

#121 - Leg Spread 3

TARGET MUSCLE(S): Hamstrings, Adductors, Erector Spinae

PROCEDURE: While you are sitting on the floor, spread your legs as wide as comfortably possible. Keep your abs firm and your head down while you reach for your toes (pointed up) or as far as possible (without creating pain).

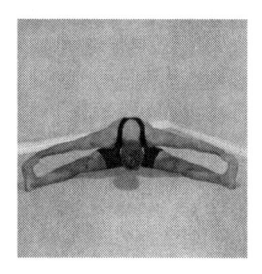

#122 - Bent Over

TARGET MUSCLE(S): Erector Spinae, Hamstrings

PROCEDURE: Gently bend over while keeping your legs straight and try to touch your toes. If you have any kind of lower back tenderness, you might try bending over using only your upper body weight to avoid being too aggressive. Try not to jerk forward to alleviate any potential discomfort to the lower back. The objective is to place your palms flat on the surface, over time.

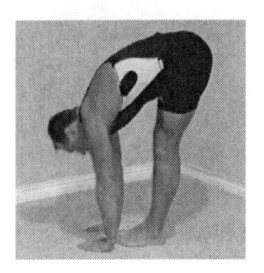

#123 - Hurdler

TARGET MUSCLE(S): Adductors, Hamstrings, Erector Spinae, Obliques

PROCEDURE: Picture an Olympic Hurdler running hurdles. This stretch involves that position except it is executed on the surface (Figure #1). Extend one of your legs so that it remains flat on the surface. Try to maintain a 90 degree angle at the hip and knee of your bent leg while keeping it on the surface. The foot of your extended leg should be pointed upward to enhance the stretch for the hamstring. Ultimately, try to bring your nose to your knee (Figure #1). Always ensure you switch sides before moving onto another stretch.

In the hurdlers position you can also reach forward with both hands and grasp the foot, ankle, knee or upper part of the leg (depending on your comfort level) and gently pull the upper body towards the leg (Figure #2).

There are a numerous variations to this stretch to challenge the adductors and hamstrings as shown in Figure #3 and the lower back/obliques as shown in Figure #4.

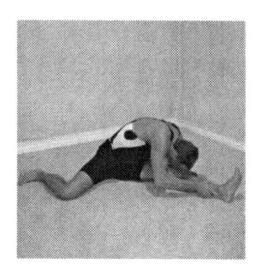

Figure #1

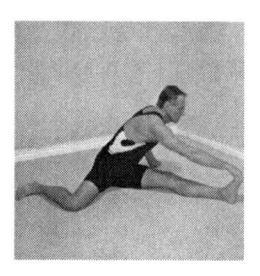

Figure #2

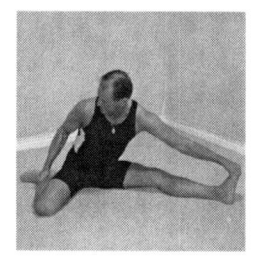

Figure #3

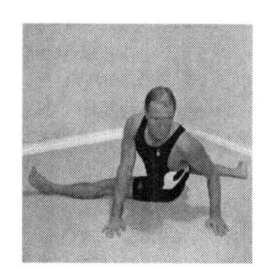

Figure #4

#124 - Straddle Leg (Advanced)

TARGET MUSCLE(S): Glutes, Hamstrings

PROCEDURE: While you are sitting, grasp the outside of one of your feet with your opposite hand. Extend your leg and pull the foot inward as shown in Figure #1. Once your leg is straight it can be crossed over, to the same side you are pulling towards with your arm, for an enhanced stretch.

It is important for this stretch that you maintain a fully extended position with your leg. The stretch will not be effective if your leg is bent. If it is difficult for you to straighten your leg try to hold on to it at a lower point (Figure #2) until enough flexibility is gained to grasp the foot (this will take practice).

This is also a very effective stretch for the IT Band which extends from the hip to your knee on the outside of your leg.

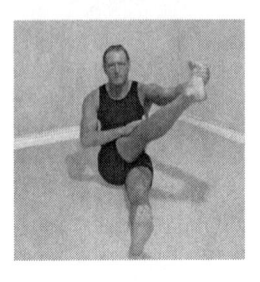

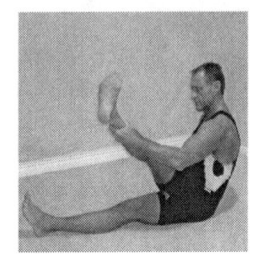

Figure #1

Figure #2

#125 - Reverse Crab – Single Leg

TARGET MUSCLE(S): Hamstrings, Adductors, Quads, Abs

PROCEDURE: Lie face down on the surface and grasp one foot with both hands while keeping your other leg extended as shown below. Gently pull your foot towards your back for an enhanced stretch.

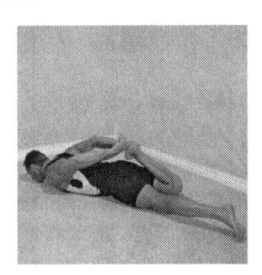

#126 - Wide Leg Squat Extension

TARGET MUSCLE(S): Adductors, Hamstrings

PROCEDURE: Stand upright and bend one knee 90 degrees while extending your opposite leg to the side. Keep the toes of your extended leg pointed upward (Figure #1). An advanced variation of this stretch involves placing your elbow, which is on the same side as the bent knee, against that knee to hold it over the heel. At the same time, try to place your opposite forearm flat, or as close as possible, on the surface (Figure #2).

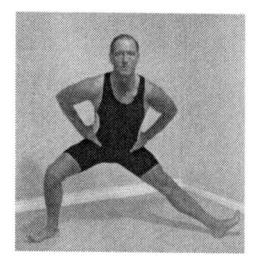

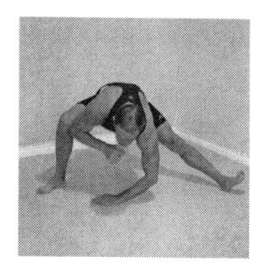

Figure #1

Figure #2

#127 - Open Leg Extension (Advanced)

TARGET MUSCLE(S): Adductors, Hamstrings

PROCEDURE: Lie down with your shoulders flat on the surface and arms laterally extended. Extend one of your legs from your body so that 90 degrees is maintained between them as shown in Figure #1. To enhance the stretch you could grasp your foot and pull it up while keeping your other leg extended with your toes pointed upward (Figure #2).

NOTE: If you want to work your glutes, raise your laterally extended leg from the surface and push through your heel of both legs to maintain the stretch (Figure #2). For this exercise, try to hold for 3-6 seconds each rep and rest 2-3 seconds between reps/sets. Complete 6-10 reps.

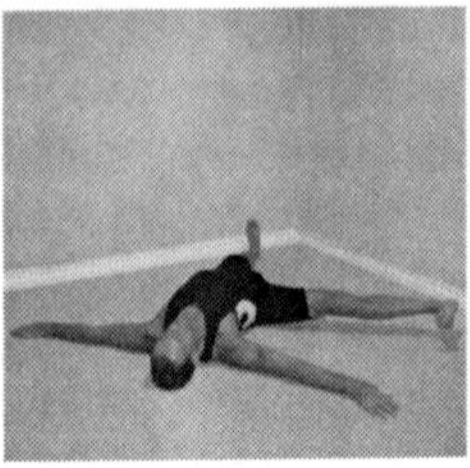

Figure #1

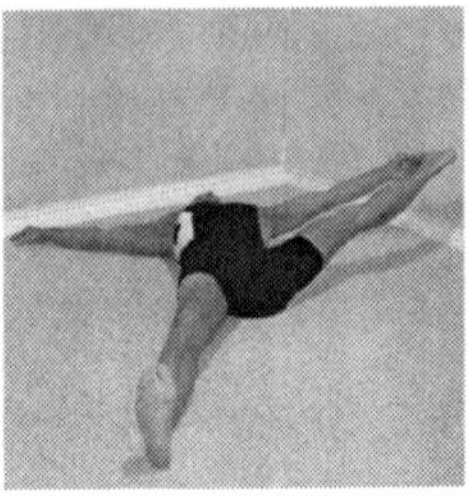

Figure #2

#128 - Praying Frog

TARGET MUSCLE(S): Adductors, Glutes

PROCEDURE: In a proper squat position spread your legs apart as wide as comfortably possible while trying to keep your knees and hips at 90 degrees. Keep your feet flat on the surface and try to push your knees out over your heels with your hands in a praying position (notice the straight line made with the forearms). Try to keep your back straight (looking up will help).

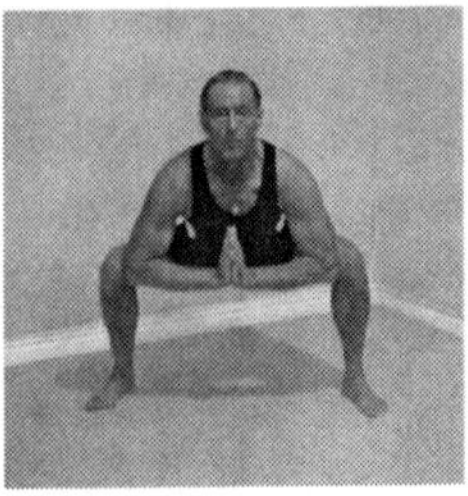

#129 - Chair Leg Extension

TARGET MUSCLE(S): Adductors, Hamstrings, Hip Flexors, Glutes

PROCEDURE: Extend both of your legs and place one of them over the back of a stable chair or couch so that your leg is 90 degrees to your body. Try to maintain your toes of the "chair" leg pointed up to assist with the stretch (Figure #1). If you would like to enhance this stretch you could bend the knee of your support leg (Figure #2). Another option is to try and touch the surface with your hand that is on the chair side as shown in Figure #3.

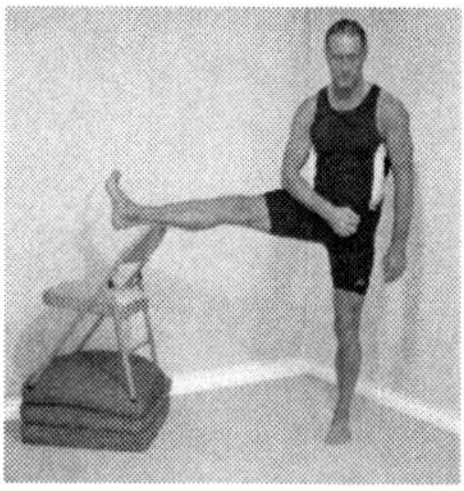

Figure #1

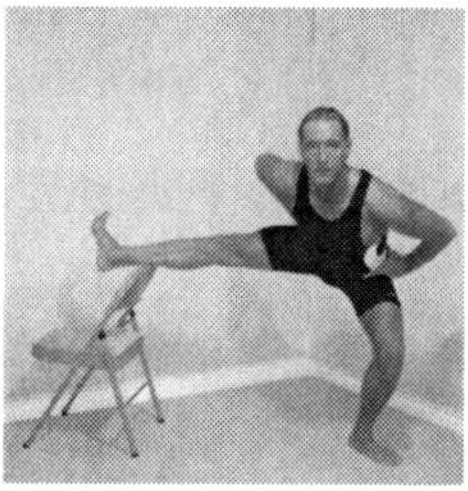

Figure #2

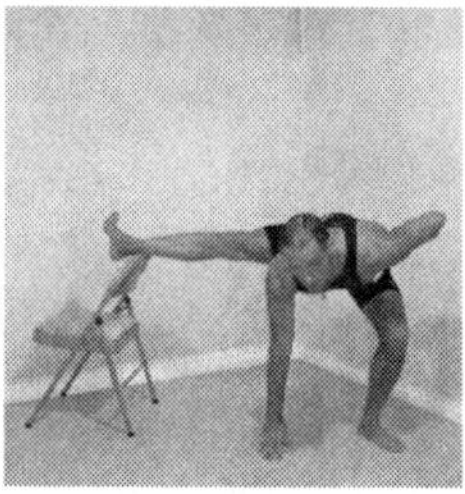

Figure #3

#130 - Seated Groin

TARGET MUSCLE(S): Groin, Adductors

PROCEDURE: Sit upright and bring your feet together. Hold onto your feet while you place your elbows against your knees. Lift your feet up while you push down on your knees with your elbows. Keep your back straight.

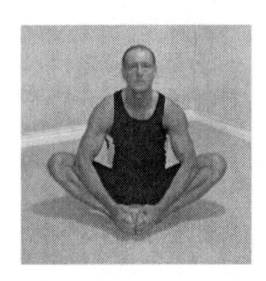

#131 - Lunge Stretch

TARGET MUSCLE(S): Psoas (muscle located near the hip/femur joints)

PROCEDURE: Assume the lunge position except this time rest your back knee on the surface. Initially, keep your front knee over your heel and your body upright. To enhance the stretch you could gradually move your knee forward and/or extend your back leg further.

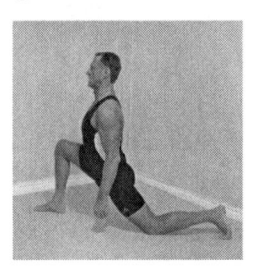

#132 - Crossover

TARGET MUSCLE(S): Adductors, Glutes

PROCEDURE: While you sit upright, extend one leg and rest the foot of your other leg over your extended knee. Reach forward and grasp the toes of your extended leg with the arm that is on the same side. Apply gentle downward pressure on your knee, with the other hand, if you would like to enhance the stretch.

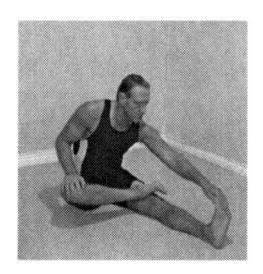

#133 - Leg Cross

TARGET MUSCLE(S): Glutes, Adductors, Quads

PROCEDURE: Lie on your back and cross your left leg over your right knee. You may enhance your stretch by applying gentle pressure with your hand to your left knee as shown in Figure #1.

An effective but advanced variation of this exercise involves the same approach as above except that you vertically extend your leg that is still on the surface while you hold onto your toes with the hand from the same side (Figure #2).

A final variation of this stretch starts off as shown in Figure #1. This time you slip the arm on your elevated bent leg side through the hole created by crossing your legs and grasp the shin of the leg that is on the surface. Take your opposite hand and place it on the outside of your "surface leg" over your other hand that is already on your shin (Figure #3). Finally, pull your shin towards your body.

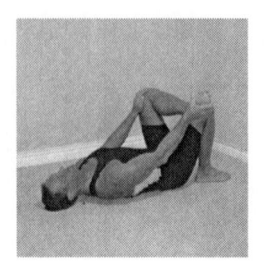

Figure #1

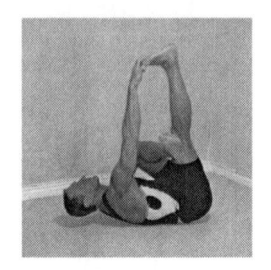

Figure #2

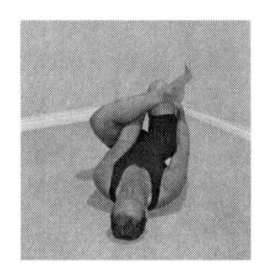

Figure #3

#134 - Ankle Reach

TARGET MUSCLE(S): Hamstrings, Glutes, Delts, Obliques

PROCEDURE: In the erect position, laterally extend both of your legs as wide as comfortably possible. Reach to one side with both hands and place them on the outside of your ankle as shown. You may need to start with reaching to the knee and work down towards your ankle over time.

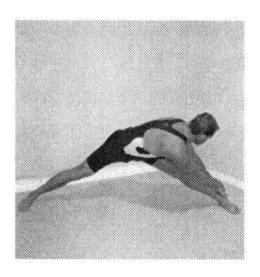

#135 - Stork

TARGET MUSCLE(S): Quads

PROCEDURE: In the erect position, bend one leg behind you and grasp your foot (touch a wall/chair for balance if you feel the need). Keep your knees together and gently hold your foot close to your buttocks (see below) until a stretch is felt on the front of your leg (quad). Tuck your pelvis in and maintain an erect position. You can slightly bend your opposite knee to assist with balance. If you have challenges with your balance, you can lie on your side and follow the same procedure.

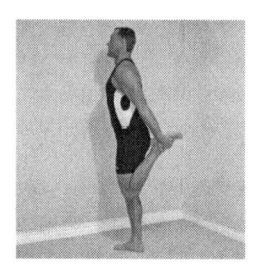

#136 - Seiza

TARGET MUSCLE(S): Quads

PROCEDURE: Sit with your knees together and your toes curled back as shown below. Lean back while keeping your back straight and make sure you keep your toes curled. This is also a good position to utilize while executing some upper body exercises like shoulder circles or arm pulls.

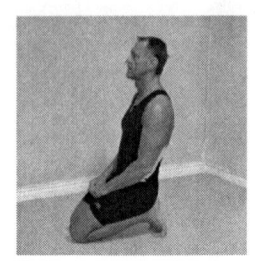

#137 - Knee to the Wall (Advanced)

TARGET MUSCLE(S) & JOINTS: Quads, Ankles

PROCEDURE: This stretch typically takes some practice. Start with the same procedure as Seiza with your back as close to the wall as possible. Bend one of your knees and place it in the corner of the floor and wall while you put both of your palms flat on the floor. Ensure that the foot of your bent knee is pointed upward (Figure #1).

To enhance your stretch you can bring your knee up from the floor while keeping your palms on the knee (Figure #2). Try to move your body upright so that it is parallel with the wall.

To enhance this stretch even further, you can try holding your back and head against the wall and even extend your arms shoulder height against the wall as well (Figure #3).

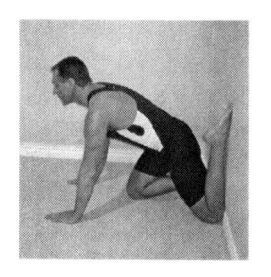

Figure #1

Figure #2

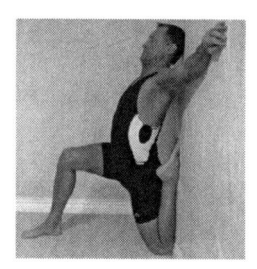

Figure #3

#138 - Crazy Pigeon (Advanced)

TARGET MUSCLE(S): Glutes, Quads

PROCEDURE: In the downward facing "Dog Pose" that was covered previously (both legs extended and hips elevated so that your body and legs are approximately 90 degrees to one another - Figure #1) bring one leg forward and curl it under your upright body while you rest on both of your arms as shown in Figure #2.

If the first step above is not enough of a stretch you can reach forward with both arms while you touch your nose to the surface as shown in Figure #3.

If you would like an even further stretch, you can go back to Figure #2. While you keep one of your legs curled under your body, bend your opposite leg up while you reach back with your arm on that same side and grasp your foot. Reach forward with your other arm, as far as possible, while gently pulling on the leg you are holding (try to keep your nose to the surface) as shown in Figure #4.

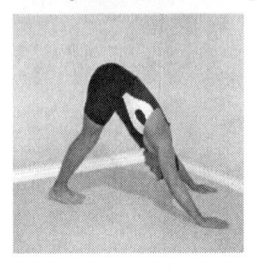

Figure #1

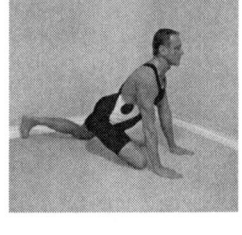

Figure #2

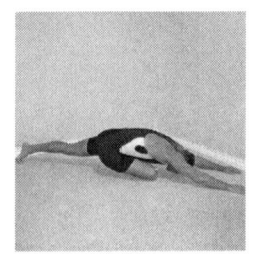

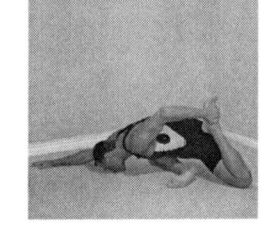

Figure #3

Figure #4

#139 - Scooping Push Up (Double Stretch)

TARGET MUSCLE(S): Glutes, Hamstrings, Pecs, Erector Spinae, Delts, Abs

PROCEDURE: Position your body as you would for the Scooping Push Up. There are two key stretch positions as shown below. The first stretch is a more relaxed position, as in the "Dog Pose", shown in Figure #1. Try to keep your head down between your shoulders for this first exercise.

For the second stretch, lower your hips and bring your abdomen as close to the surface as possible without touching. Your arms and legs remain laterally extended (partially) and do not move from the previous stretch performed. You look up as high as you possibly can (only your feet and hands touch the surface) to enhance the stretch while holding the position as shown in Figure #2.

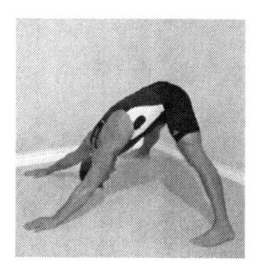

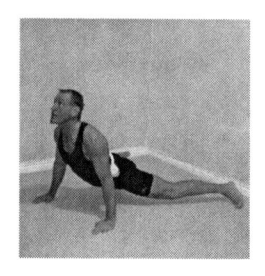

Figure #1

Figure #2

#140 - Marry Me

TARGET MUSCLE(S): Hip Flexors, Glutes, Erector Spinae, Obliques

PROCEDURE: While you kneel down on one knee, keep your other knee at a 90 degree angle so your quads are level with the surface as shown in Figure #1. To intensify the stretch, and engage your obliques, you can raise your arms shoulder level and twist your upper body 90 degrees or more as shown in Figure #2. A further stretch could involve bending down from your position in Figure #2 so that your elbows touch the surface as shown in Figure #3.

Figure #1

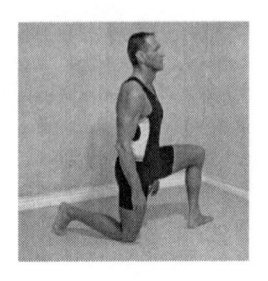

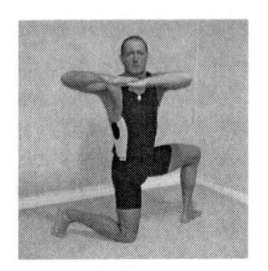

Figure #2

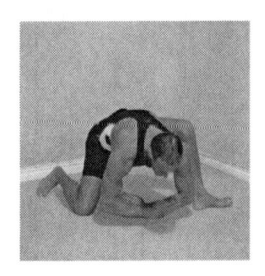

Figure #3

#141 - Calf

TARGET MUSCLE(S): Calves, Achilles

PROCEDURE: In the downward facing "Dog Pose", as shown in Figure #1, alternate raising your heels off the surface while your opposite foot is flat on the surface.

Another version of this stretch involves your feet placed about 75-100mm (3-4 inches) apart and 750-1000mm (3-4 feet) away from the wall. Ensure your glutes remain tucked in and your back straight while you try to place your feet flat on the surface and then raise them as high as possible (Figure #2).

To stretch the Achilles tendon, execute the stretch shown in Figure #2 and alternate bending your knee slightly, as shown in Figure #3, while you gradually lift your heel from the surface and hold for 3-5 seconds.

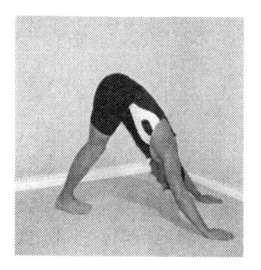

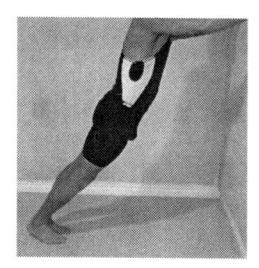

Figure #1

Figure #2

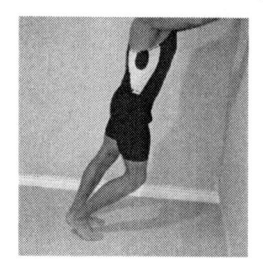

Figure #3

B. UPPER BODY

#142 - Back Scratch

TARGET MUSCLE(S): Triceps

PROCEDURE: As shown below, reach back over your shoulder with one arm while holding a towel. Use your opposite arm to grasp the towel and gently pull down to create the stretch.

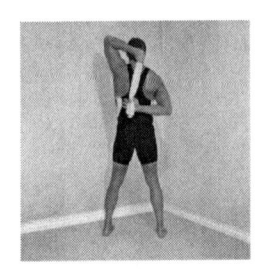

#143 - About Face

TARGET MUSCLE(S): Biceps, Pecs, Delts

PROCEDURE: Place your body perpendicular to a wall with your arm extended shoulder height behind you and your palm placed flat against the wall (thumb pointed up). Keep your arm and the entire side of your body (from foot to shoulder – **especially the shoulder**) against the wall. Turn your head (face) away from the wall as far as possible to maximize the stretch (Figure #1).

Another version of this stretch involves lying down on your side so that it is perpendicular with the surface. Your floor side arm is extended behind you, shoulder level (palm facing down) as shown in Figure #2. You can intensify the stretch by extending your upper leg forward and your upper arm back as shown.

Figure #1   Figure #2

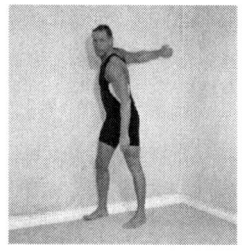

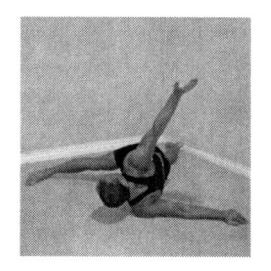

#144 - Thumbs Down

TARGET MUSCLE(S): Biceps

PROCEDURE: In the erect position, laterally extend your arms while you turn your thumbs down. For a greater stretch you could try to push your arms back while maintaining this position.

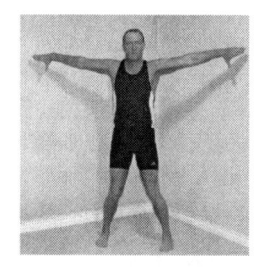

#145 - Front Shoulder Pull

TARGET MUSCLE(S): Delts

PROCEDURE: Maintain square shoulders with your body and extend one of your arms shoulder height and across your chest. Use your opposite arm to grasp your elbow and gently pull it inward to get the stretch.

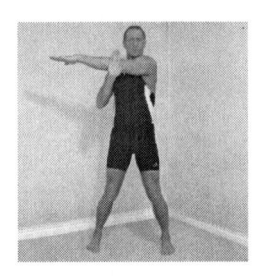

#146 - Back Shoulder Pull

TARGET MUSCLE(S): Delts

PROCEDURE: This is similar in approach to the Front Shoulder Pull. The difference is that with the arm that comes across your chest, reach back as if to scratch your back and grasp the elbow with your opposite hand. Pull the elbow in towards your body and pull even further with the hand that is reaching behind your back.

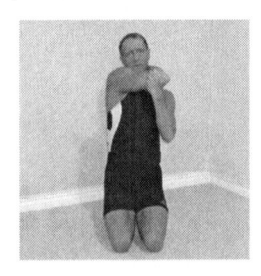

#147 - Shoulder Reach

TARGET MUSCLE(S): Delts

PROCEDURE: In the erect position, face a wall and vertically extend your arm while keeping your entire body against the wall as shown below. When you release from the stretch, gently lower your arm laterally while maintaining body contact with the wall. A variation of this stretch involves placing the entire side of your body against the wall.

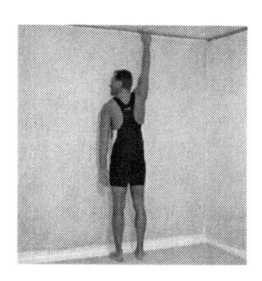

#148 - Duck Wings

TARGET MUSCLE(S): Delts

PROCEDURE: In the erect position, keep your shoulders square with your body while bending your elbows and reaching back with them as shown below.

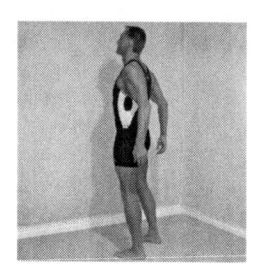

#149 - Worship

TARGET MUSCLE(S): Lats, Delts, Erector Spinae, Quads

PROCEDURE: Kneel down on the surface with the tops of your feet on the floor. Extend your arms above your head and then bend towards the surface as shown below. Place your palms flat on the surface and try to keep your nose down as low as possible.

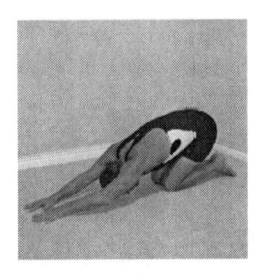

#150 - Trap/Neck Sqeeze

TARGET MUSCLE(S): Trapezius, Neck Muscles

PROCEDURE: Keep your shoulders square with your body and tilt your head laterally while trying to bring your ear as close to your shoulder as possible (hold for 3-5 seconds and alternate from side to side 6 times each side). To enhance the stretch you could tilt your head forward while moving side to side. Do not be surprised if you feel some "cracking" or loosening of the joints.

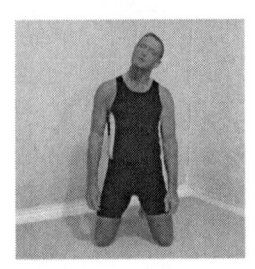

#151- Reverse Handshake

TARGET MUSCLE(S): Pecs

PROCEDURE: Bring one hand to your side as if you were returning it from executing a punch. Your palm should face up. Bring your other hand behind your back and clasp the other hand so that they are palm to palm as shown below. Try to squeeze your elbows as close together as possible. Repeat the exercise on the other side.

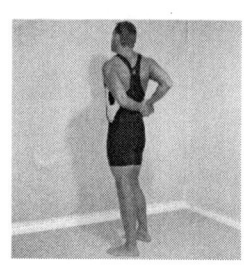

#152 - Pec Sqeeze

TARGET MUSCLE(S): Pecs, Delts

PROCEDURE: Maintain the erect position (do not bend over) and clasp your hands behind your back while keeping them in the extended position (or as best you can). Try to squeeze your elbows together as shown below and raise your arms to enhance the stretch.

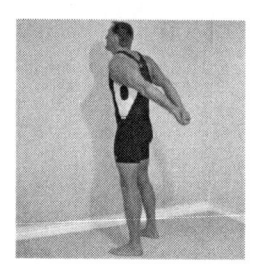

#153 - Hug Yourself

TARGET MUSCLE(S): Rhomboids

PROCEDURE: Square your shoulders with your body and wrap both arms around yourself while reaching, as best you can, to grasp each opposite shoulder. Always try to reach further.

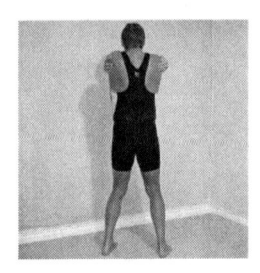

#154 - Wrist Extensor/Flexor

TARGET MUSCLE GROUP: Wrists, Forearms

PROCEDURE: Use a flat surface, like a wall, and place the back of your hand flat and downward against the surface as shown in Figure #1 for an extensor stretch. Place your palm flat and upward against the surface, as shown in Figure #2, for a flexor stretch.

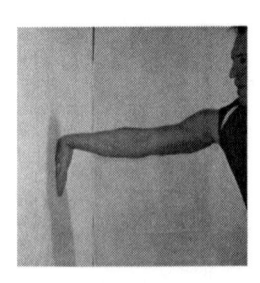

Figure #1 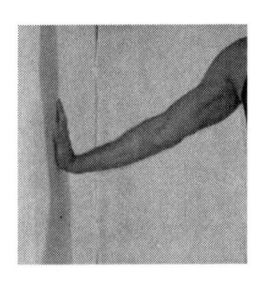   Figure #2

C. ABS, BACK & NECK

#155 - Prone

TARGET MUSCLE(S): Abs, Erector Spinae

PROCEDURE: Lie face down on the surface and lean on your elbows while staying on your toes as shown. Keep your core (abs and obliques) tight and back straight.

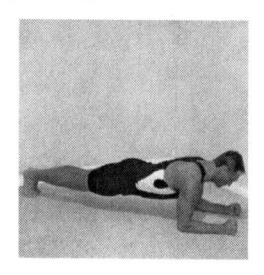

#156 - Pretzel

TARGET MUSCLE(S): Abs, Obliques

PROCEDURE: While sitting down, bend one of your legs at the knee and rest it on the surface. Place your other foot on the outside of your "surface knee" as shown in Figure #1. Place your opposite elbow on the outside of the upright knee and reach around behind you with your other arm as far as possible as shown in Figure #2. Turn your head to face your backside (same side as the arm that is reaching behind) to enhance the stretch.

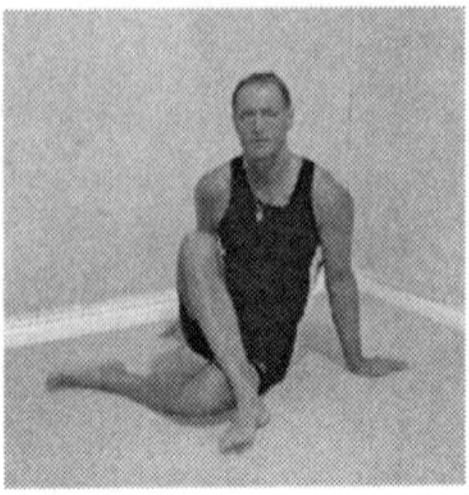

Figure #1

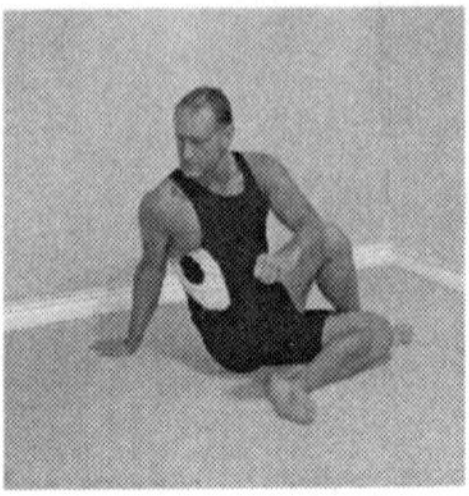

Figure #2

#157 - Cobra

TARGET MUSCLE(S): Erector Spinae, Abs

PROCEDURE: In the Standard Push Up position, straighten your arms so that they are extended while your legs remain flat on the surface as shown in Figure #1. Look up as high as possible to enhance your stretch. To take the stretch a step further, you can come up on your toes allowing your mid section to sink lower.

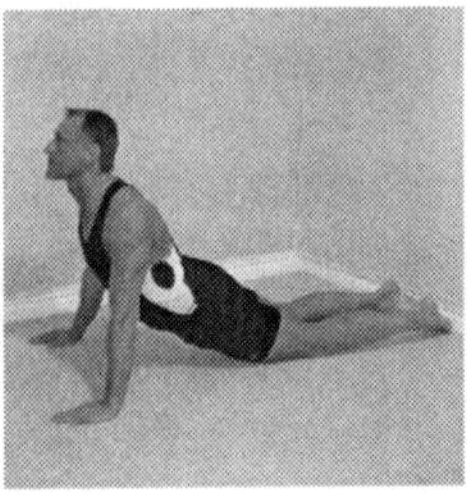

#158 - Reverse Crab — Double Leg

TARGET MUSCLE(S): Abs, Quads

PROCEDURE: Lie face down on the surface and grasp you feet or ankles. Gently pull your legs in towards you while you look up as high as possible.

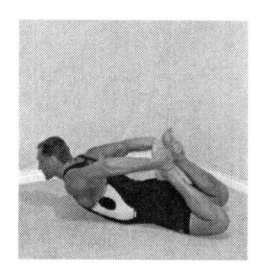

#159 - Mad Cat

TARGET MUSCLE(S): Erector Spinae

PROCEDURE: In the kneeling position, extend your arms and round out your spine as shown below. Try to keep your abs tight and head tucked in.

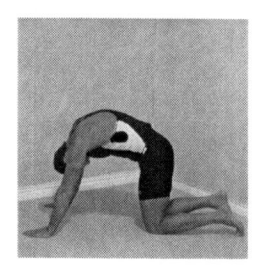

#160 - Roller Ball

TARGET MUSCLE(S): Erector Spinae

PROCEDURE: Lie on your back and bring your knees into your chest. Wrap both arms around the legs as shown below and pull your legs in tight to your body. A variation of this stretch is to roll back and forth on the curvature of your back like a rocking chair and/or side to side.

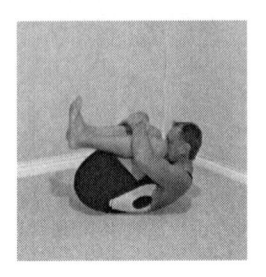

#161 - Lower Body Twist

TARGET MUSCLE(S): Erector Spinae, Obliques, Glutes

PROCEDURE: Lie down with your arms extended laterally while you raise both of your knees so they are approximately 90 degrees to your body. Keep your knees together and your arms/shoulders flat on the surface as shown below.

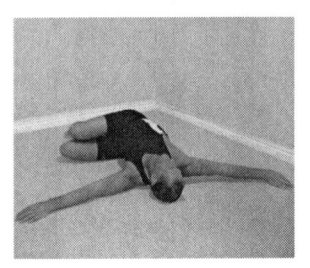

#162 - Stick Man

TARGET MUSCLE(S): Erector Spinae, Adductors

PROCEDURE: Lie face down with your arms extended shoulder level. Keep your arms pinned to the surface while you laterally extend one of your legs to a point where it touches your hand.

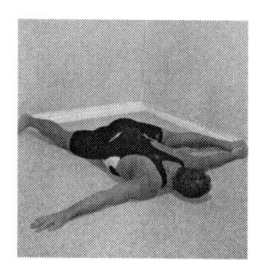

#163 – Lower Back (Advanced)

TARGET MUSCLE(S): Erector Spinae, Glutes

PROCEDURE: Lie on your back and bring one leg up so that your quad is 90 degrees to your body and knee bent. One of your arms remains shoulder level and the other you can use to pull your leg towards you for an enhanced stretch. You can also raise your head and your extended leg to engage your abs.

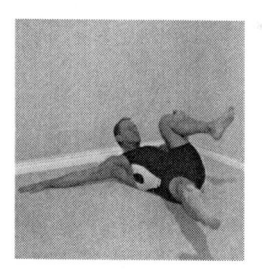

#164 – Back Challenge

TARGET MUSCLE(S): Erector Spinae

PROCEDURE: Lie face down with your arms laterally extended shoulder level and your legs laterally extended as far as possible. While you maintain extended legs and arms, raise your legs and/or arms from the surface as shown below.

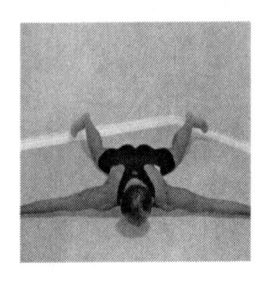

#165 - Side Bend 1

TARGET MUSCLE(S): Obliques

PROCEDURE: Sit on the floor with your legs crossed and arms extended above your head. Clasp your hands together and reach to one side of your body as far as you can while keeping your body straight. Ensure you maintain extended arms while bending only at your waist as shown below.

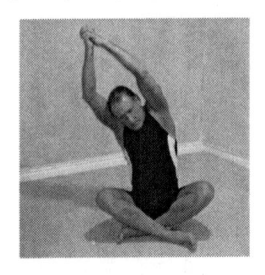

#166 - Side Bend 2

TARGET MUSCLE(S): Obliques

PROCEDURE: Extend your legs slightly to your side while extending one arm above your head. In the meantime, reach down with the other arm. Gently reach 3 times with both arms before repeating on the other side (see below). Bend your knee on the side you are reaching down to and try to reach a little further each time with both arms.

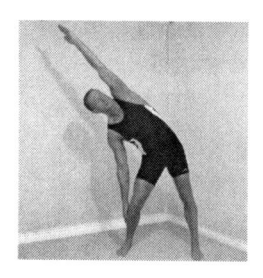

#167 - Torso Bend

TARGET MUSCLE(S): Obliques

PROCEDURE: In the erect position, extend your arms and clasp your hands together straight above your head. Try to keep your abs tight while you lean to your side 3 times. Slightly bend your knee on the side you are leaning as shown below. Repeat on the other side. For an additional stretch, you can hold a water bottle above your head.

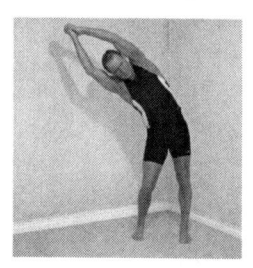

#168 – Glute Bend

TARGET MUSCLE(S): Obliques, Glutes, Hamstrings

PROCEDURE: This is effectively the same as the previous stretch. The difference is that your legs are laterally extended as far as comfortably possible (try to maintain them extended while bending to your side). In doing so, the glutes and hamstrings will be introduced into the stretch. Try to keep tight abs while you lean to your side 3 times before repeating on your other side.

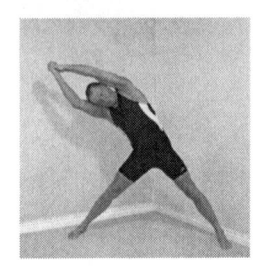

#169 - Full Body

TARGET MUSCLE(S): Erector Spinae, Abs, Obliques, Pecs, Quads, Hamstrings, Delts, Biceps

PROCEDURE: Stand erect with your legs and arms laterally extended as far as comfortably possible. Lean back as far as you can as shown in Figure #1 and #2.

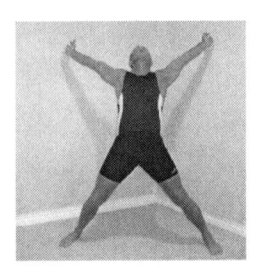

Figure #1

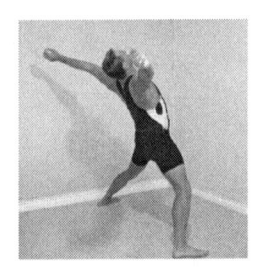

Figure #2

#170 - Neck Stretch

TARGET MUSCLE(S): Splenius Cervicis, Levator Scapulae, Scalene, Sternocleidomastoid

PROCEDURE: Lean your head laterally to one side while you gently press with your hand to increase the stretch (Figure #1). Hold for a count of 6 and repeat on the other side. Repeat this procedure by pushing your chin into your chest and leaning back (while applying pressure with your hands) as far as possible while holding for the same count (Figure #2). Perform the same steps leaning back with your neck and applying forward pressure with your hands.

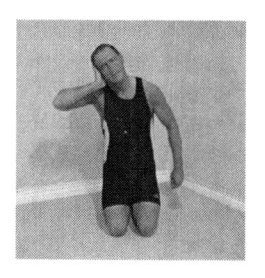

Figure #1

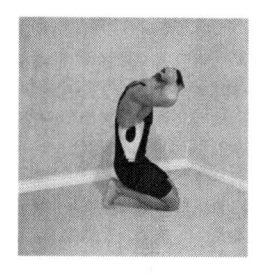

Figure #2

SAMPLE PROGRAMS

Now that you have been introduced to a number of exercises and drills, the focus of this chapter is to provide you with guidance so you may incorporate them into your individual fitness program using many different training disciplines. Before creating your own program, I recommend you try some of the sample programs which follow. That way you can gain an appreciation of their structure, degree of difficulty and the benefits they provide.

Although each of the programs in this section follows a specific format, there are no specific individual exercises that must be included in each program. For example, you can substitute a standard push up with a tiger eye push up or replace a front lunge with a rotating lunge. And of course your exercises will change over time with enhanced fitness. **The exercises included in the programs are simply intended to provide you with some ideas.** You may also want to vary the programs to create different types of workouts. I really encourage you to keep changing exercises around once you gain a level of comfort and familiarity with them and the sample programs. Just remember, it is important to keep challenging your body with change.

Typically, the sample programs provide for a full body workout, with the exception of the running drills that are more cardiovascular in nature and the 10 Minute Office Program that is simply a "health break". Some of the programs are designed specifically to serve as a substitute for a regularly scheduled workout simply to add variety and challenge. They all draw from the numerous exercises and training methodologies provided within this guide.

The following programs have been tested by individuals with varying degrees of fitness and should be appropriate to get you started. However, you should consider your own requirements, goals and level of fitness, before trying them, and make necessary adjustments to the exercises and programs as required.

Some of the sample programs, in terms of exercise content, may not seem an appropriate match for you based on your present level of fitness. You will need to assess your fitness level and determine what is best for you in terms of the number of exercises, reps and sets you chose initially. Because you will be able to ramp up your program content over time as your fitness level improves, there shouldn't be any limitations to your progress.

There are programs for the Beginner, Intermediate and Advanced levels of fitness. The sample programs also apply many of the approaches covered earlier, including Shock Treatment, Mixing, Stacking, Pyramiding, Enhanced Reps and, Circuit and Interval Training. An important principle to keep in mind with these types of programs and training is that when you get to a higher level of fitness the program content, reps, sets and other aspects of your exercises and drills should change. You may also want to vary the exercises and drills so the body is always kept off guard – remember there is "no norm".

Sample "Full Body" Beginner Program

Work out days - Mon/Wed/Fri OR Tues/Thurs/Sat
Approximate duration – 25-35 minutes

	set x reps	exercise/drill
WARM UP		Neck #1
	1x5	Leg Circles #9
	1x5	Shoulder Circles #3
	1x5	Torso Rotation #7
	1x10	Hip Twist #5
	2-3 minutes	Spot Jog #15
CARDIO	5 minutes	Run, Cycle, Climb Stairs
	1x12	Jumping Jacks #86
	5 minutes	Spot Jog, Run, Cycle, or Climb Stairs

RESISTANCE TRAINING

Lower Body	1x10	Standard Squat #28
	1x10	Lunge #22
	1x10	Bum Burner Bent Leg #37
	1x6	Bum Burner Extension #38
	1x8	Bum Burner Kick #39
	1x12	Toe Raise #43
Upper Body	1x5	Standard Push Up #44
	1x5	Dip #55
	1x5	Shoulder Push Up #49
	1x10	Arm Pull #56
	1x20	Punch Drill #100
	1x10	Upper Cut Drill #102

Abs & Obliques	1x10	Sit Up #59
	1x10	Leg Raise #60
	1x20	Body Twist #68

COOL DOWN & STRETCHING (20-30 seconds each)

Lower Body
- Stork #135
- Leg Splits #117
- Bent Over #122
- Hurdler #123
- Calf #141

Upper Body
- About Face #143
- Thumbs Down #144
- Back Scratch #142

Abs, Obliques, & Back
- Prone #155
- Side Bend 1 #165

Sample "Full Body" Intermediate Program

Work out days - Mon/Wed/Fri OR Tues/Thurs/Sat
Approximate duration – 35-60 minutes

	set x reps	exercise/drill
WARM UP		Neck #1
	1X10	Leg Circles #9
	1x10	Shoulder Circles #3
	3-5 minutes	Spot Jog #15
	1x10	Cross Crawl #11
CARDIO	3x6 minutes	Spot Run #17
	3x12	Jumping Jacks #86
	3x10	Front Kick Drill #107
	3x5	Combo Punch Drill #106
	3x5	Karaoke #98
RESISTANCE TRAINING		
Lower Body	1x15	Standard Squat #28
	1x15	Bum Burner Bent Leg #37
	1x15	Bum Burner Extension #38
	1x15	Bum Burner Kick #39
	1x15	Lunge #22
	1x15	Bum Burner Hold #40
	1x15	Bum Burner Circle #41
	1x15	Rotating Lunge #24
	1x20	Toe Raise #43
Upper Body	1x12	Standard Push Up #44
	1x12	Shoulder Push Up #49
	2x15	Arm Pull #56
	2x20	Power Punch Drill #103
	2x20	Upper Cut Drill #102
	2x12	Dip #55
	2x10	Wrist Rolls #58

NOTE: Each push up set above is followed by one set of each exercise #56 through #58 inclusive.

	1x6	Tiger Eye Push Up #48
Abs/Obliques	1x20	Bicycle #69
	1x20	Sit Up #59
	1x20	Body Twist #68
	1x20	Ab Crunch #74
	1x20	Leg Raise #60

COOL DOWN & STRETCHING (20-30 seconds each)

Lower Body
- Stork #135
- Straddle Leg #124
- Single Vertical Leg #118
- Leg Spread 2 #120
- Praying Frog #128
- Leg Cross #133

Upper Body
- About Face #143
- Back Shoulder Pull #146
- Thumbs Down #144
- Back Scratch #142
- Duck Wings #148

Abs, Obliques & Back
- Prone #155
- Pretzel #156
- Cobra #157
- Side Bend 1 #165
- Full Body #169

Sample "Full Body" Advanced Program

Work out days - Mon/Tues/Thurs/Fri OR Tues/Wed/Fri/Sat
Approximate duration – 45-75 minutes

	set x reps	exercise/drill
WARM UP		Neck #1
	3-5 minutes	Spot Jog #15
	1X10	Leg Circles #9
	1x10	Shoulder Circles #3
	See exercise	Integrated Shoulder #4
	See exercise	Integrated Torso #6
	See exercise	Integrated Hip #10
	1x10	Extended Kick #12
	1x10	Cross Crawl #11
CARDIO	3x5 minutes	Stair Climb #16
	3x10	Upper Cut Drill #102
	3x15	Kick Combo Drill #113
	3x20 sec.	Spot Run #17
	3x10	Line Drill #116

NOTE: Complete one set of all exercises #16 through #116 inclusive and rest 20 sec. before the next set

RESISTANCE TRAINING

Lower Body	1x15	Adductor Leg Raise #34
	2x15	Lunge #22
	2x15	Bum Burner Bent Leg #37
	2x15	Bum Burner Extension #38
	2x15	Bum Burner Kick #39
	2x15	Bum Burner Hold #40
	2x15	Bum Burner Circle #41

NOTE: Complete 1 set of exercises #22 through #41 and repeat before moving to the next exercise

	3x6	Burpee's #97
	3x10	Jump Squat #89

NOTE: Complete exercise #97 & #89 and rest for 15 sec. before repeating

	1x20	Toe Raise #43
Upper Body	3x10	Standard Push Up #44
	3x10	Shoulder Push Up #49
	3x6	Tiger Eye Push Up #48
	3x6	Scooping Push Up #52
	3x15	Dip #55
	3x15	Arm Pull #56
	3x20	Combo Punch Drill #106

NOTE: Complete 1 set of exercise #44 through #106 and repeat

	1x10	Perfect Push Up #50
	3x20	Upper Cut Drill #102
	2x10	Wrist Roll #58
Abs/Obliques	2x15	Bicycle #69
	2x15	Sit Up #59
	2x15	Body Twist #68
	2x15	Ab Crunch #74
	2x15	Oblique Twist #83
	2x15	Leg Raise #60
	2x10	Boomerang #73
	1x20	3 Way Ab Plank #85
		Prone #84 (20-30 sec)

COOL DOWN & STRETCHING (20-30 seconds each)

Lower Body	Upper Body	Abs, Obliques & Back
Stork #135	About Face #143	Lower Body Twist #161
Leg Splits #117	Shoulder Reach #147	Roller Ball #160
Leg Spread 1 #119	Worship #149	Cobra #157
Leg Spread 3 #121	Back Shoulder Pull #146	Full Body #169
Chair Leg Extension #129	Thumbs Down #144	Back Challenge #164
Ankle Reach #134	Back Scratch #142	
Leg Cross #133		
Crazy Pigeon #138		
Seiza #136		

Sample
"Shock Treatment/Fat Burner" Program

Work out days – a substitute for any normal workout
Duration – 45-75 minutes - depends on fitness level

	set x reps	exercise/drill
WARM UP		Neck #1
	1X10	Leg Circles #9
	1x10	Shoulder Circles #3
	See exercise	Integrated Shoulder #4
	See exercise	Integrated Torso #6
	See exercise	Integrated Hip #10
	1x10	Toe Touch #8
	3-5 minutes	Spot Jog #15
RESISTANCE TRAINING		
Abs/Obliques	2x10	Boomerang #73
	2x15	Leg Raise #60
	2x15	Body Twist #68
	2x15	Ab Crunch #74
	2x15	Oblique Twist #83
	2x15	Sit Up #59
	2x10	Bicycle #69
	1x20	3 Way Ab Plank #85
		Prone #84 (20-30 sec)
Upper Body	3x10	Standard Push Up #44
	3x10	Clap Push Up #45
	3x6	Tiger Eye Push Up #48
	3x6	Scooping Push Up #52
	3x15	Dip #55
	3x10	Shoulder Push Up #49
	3x15	Arm Pull #56

NOTE: Complete one set of all exercises #44 through #56 inclusive and rest 20 sec. before starting the next set

	1x6	Side Push Up #53
	2x10	Wrist Roll each way #58
CARDIO	4x3 minutes	Stair Climb #16
	4x10	Shadow Spar Drill #115

	4x10	Kick Combo Drill #113
	4x20 sec.	Spot Run #17
	4x10	Combo Punch Drill #106

RESISTANCE TRAINING

Lower Body	1x10	Adductor Leg Raise #34
	2x15	Jump Lunge Shift #92
	2x15	Bum Burner Bent Leg #37
	2x15	Bum Burner Extension #38
	2x15	Bum Burner Kick #39
	2x15	Bum Burner Hold #40
	2x15	Bum Burner Circle #41
	3x10	Jump Squat #89
	3x6	Burpee's #97
	2x20	Toe Raise #43

COOL DOWN & STRETCHING (20-30 seconds each)

Lower Body	Stork #135
	Leg Splits #117
	Wide Leg Extension #126
	Leg Spread 1 #119
	Hurdler #123
	Crossover #132
	Scoop Push Up Stretch #139
	Lunge #131
	Knee to Wall #137
Upper Body	About Face #143
	Front Shoulder Pull #145
	Worship #149
	Back Scratch #142
	Thumbs Down #144
Abs, Obliques & Back	Torso Bend #167
	Glute Bend #168
	Back Challenge #164
	Stickman #162
	Full Body #169

Sample "Pyramid – Full Body Cardio" Program

Work out days – a substitute for any normal workout
Duration – 35-75 minutes dependant on fitness level

WARM UP

1 x 10 Leg Circles #9

Integrators #4, #6, #10

3-5 minutes - Spot Jog #15

1 x 10 Cross Crawl #11

Bottom of Pyramid

40 second Spot Run #17

18 reps Upper Cut Drill #102

15 reps Lunge each leg #22

17 reps Shoulder Push Up #49

20 reps Leg Raise #60

45 second rest

2nd

35 second Spot Run #17

16 reps Power "P" Drill #103

14 reps Std Squat #28

16 reps Std Push Up #44

20 reps Ab Crunch #74

40 second rest

3rd

30 second Spot Run #17

14 reps Combo "P" Drill #106

13 reps Lunge each leg #22

15 reps Shoulder Push Up #49

15 reps Body Twist #68

35 second rest

4th

25 second Spot Run #17

12 reps Rabbit Punch Drill #104

12 reps Std Squat #28

14 reps Std Push Up #44

15 reps Bicycle #69

30 second rest

5th

20 second Spot Run #17

10 reps Elbow Punch Drill #105

11 reps Lunge each leg #22

10 reps Scooping Push Up #52

14 reps 3 Way Ab Crunch #75

25 second rest

Top of Pyramid

15 second Spot Run #17

8 reps Punch Drill Horse #101

10 reps Std Squat #28

6 reps Tiger Eye Push Up #48

13 reps Abs - your choice

Additional levels can be added or deleted to the Pyramid consistent with fitness level. Another variation, or challenge, could involve going back to the bottom from the top, after a 20 second rest.

NOTE: For the stretching component of this program you can borrow from one of the other sample programs and vary it to suit your own needs.

Sample "Circuit" Program

Your fitness level will determine the duration of time you spend on any one exercise and the number of rounds and exercises you include. Start with 15 seconds for each exercise and increase 5 seconds as fitness level improves. Each Round places focus on different areas like the lower body, core conditioning and the upper body. Execute all the exercises in each round before moving to the next. Spot run or jog 30-90 seconds between rounds.

Duration – 20-45 minutes - depends on fitness level

WARM UP

1x10 Knee Hug #13 3-5 minutes - Spot Jog #15
1x10 Cross Crawl #11 1 x 10 Hi Step #14

1st Round 1. Lunge #22
(Lower Body) 2. Standard Squat #28
  3. Bum Burner Bent Leg #37
  4. Mountain Climb #93
  5. Front/Back Jump Lunge #91
  6. Kirtzie #99

2nd Round 1. Bicycle #69
(Core) 2. Leg Tuck #65
  3. "V" Leg Raise #61
  4. Turbo Twist #76
  5. Boomerang #73
  6. Punch Leg Raise #63

3rd Round 1. Std Push Up #44
(Upper Body) 2. Dip #55
  3. Scooping Push Up #52
  4. Arm Pull #56
  5. Tiger Eye Push Up #48
  6. Burpee's #97

NOTE: For the stretching component of this program you can borrow from one of the other sample programs and vary it to suit your own needs.

Sample "Interval" Program

This "Full Body" workout can be utilized for any level of fitness provided you make adjustments to the exercises, reps and duration that matches with your level of fitness. It's a "high impact" cardio workout that incorporates strength training. The only rest is "active rest". This example is based on an Intermediate fitness level that involves 30 seconds for each exercise.

Duration – 20-45 minutes

WARM UP

1x10 Leg Circles #9

Integrators #4, #6, #10

3-5 minutes - Spot Jog #15

1 x 10 Torso Rotation #7

1st Set

1. Shoulder Push Up #49
2. Std Squat #28
3. Jumping Jacks #86
4. Ab Crunch #74
5. Shadow Sparring #115
6. 30 sec. Run/Jog

2nd Set

1. Std Push Up #44
2. Std Lunge #22
3. Jump Squat #89
4. Leg Raise #60
5. Kirtzie #99
6. 30 sec. Run/Jog

3rd Set

1. Tiger Eye Push Up #48
2. Wide Squat #29
3. Jump Lunge-shift #92
4. Bicycle #69
5. Shadow Sparring #115
6. 30 sec. Run/Jog

4th Set

1. Scoop Push Up #52
2. Rotate Lunge #24
3. Burpees #97
4. Punch Leg Raise #63
5. Kirtzie #99
6. 30 sec. Run/Jog

5th Set

1. Tricep Push Up #46
2. Adductor Leg Raise #34
3. Split Jumping Jacks #88
4. Side Crunch #70
5. Shadow Sparring #115
6. 30 sec. Run/Jog

6th Set

1. Perfect Push Up #50
2. Duck Walk #33
3. Box Jump #90
4. Vertical Leg #64
5. Kirtzie #99
6. 30 sec. Run/Jog

NOTE: For the stretching component of the program you can borrow from the other sample programs and vary it to suit your own needs.

Sample Running Drills

The following drills could be utilized for the cardio component of a workout or even a focused cardio program. Each drill should be accompanied with a warm up and cool down (with stretching) that you can borrow from one of the appropriate sample programs provided.

NOTE: these programs are designed more for the Intermediate to Advanced levels of fitness. They can easily be toned down to suit the Beginner or even other training needs you may have. These drills can also incorporate various other exercises presented in this guide to "Mix" applications in an effort to enhance the workout or "fat burn", e.g. push ups, sit ups or block/punch/kick drills between sprints (active rest).

Simple Wind Sprints

At full speed run the distances shown and rest as shown.

	DISTANCE	REST
1.	40 metre/yard sprint	10 seconds
2.	40 metre/yard sprint	10 seconds
3.	30 metre/yard sprint	10 seconds
4.	30 metre/yard sprint	10 seconds
5.	20 metre/yard sprint	10 seconds
6.	20 metre/yard sprint	10 seconds
7.	10 metre/yard sprint	10 seconds
8.	10 metre/yard sprint	10 seconds
9.	5 metre/yard sprint	10 seconds
10.	5 metre/yard sprint	10 seconds

For an enhanced challenge run a second complete routine after a 5 minute rest starting at the beginning with the 40 yard sprint.

Mountain Climb

At full speed run the distances and rest as shown.

	DISTANCE	REST
1.	20 metre/yard sprint	10 seconds
2.	20 metre/yard sprint	10 seconds
3.	30 metre/yard sprint	15 seconds
4.	30 metre/yard sprint	15 seconds
5.	40 metre/yard sprint	20 seconds
6.	40 metre/yard sprint	20 seconds
7.	50 metre/yard sprint	25 seconds
8.	50 metre/yard sprint	25 seconds
9.	60 metre/yard sprint	30 seconds
10.	60 metre/yard sprint	30 seconds
11.	70 metre/yard sprint	35 seconds
12.	70 metre/yard sprint	35 seconds
13.	80 metre/yard sprint	40 seconds
14.	80 metre/yard sprint	40 seconds
15.	100 metre/yard sprint	50 seconds
16.	100 metre/yard sprint	50 seconds

A double Mountain Climb would involve a 5 minute rest at the top before starting again with the 100 yard sprint and climbing 'down' the Mountain.

Spot Run Challenge

This is a Spot Run Drill that involves high stepping intensity followed by rest (raise your knees to your waist while maintaining your arms shoulder height) for the times shown. When resting, you should continue to walk about for active rest until you commence the next set.

LENGTH OF REP	**REST**
1. 45 second spot run	20 seconds
2. 45 second spot run	20 seconds
3. 40 second spot run	15 seconds
4. 35 second spot run	15 seconds
5. 30 second spot run	15 seconds
6. 25 second spot run	10 seconds
7. 20 second spot run	10 seconds
8. 15 second spot run	10 seconds
9. 10 second spot run	5 seconds
10. 10 second spot run	5 seconds

For a real challenge run a second complete drill after a 5 minute rest, starting with the 10 second spot run.

The Office Program – 10 Minute Health Break

This "Full Body" health break that follows is designed to give your body a shot of energy that can break up your day and help you be more productive. These simple but effective exercises can easily be done, almost anywhere, including an office or work station.

The exercises suggested have been carefully selected to help replenish your body, and not complete an intense workout.

Loosen Up	A. 1x5 Leg Circles #9
	and/or
	B. 1x5 Shoulder Circles #3
	C. 1x3 Torso Rotation #7
	and/or
	D. 1x3 Hip Twist #5
Lower Body	A. 1x5 Standard Squat #28
	and/or
	B. 1x5 Standard Lunge #22
Upper Body	A. 1x5 Standard Push Up #44
	and/or
	B. 1x5 Dip (with a chair/desk) #55
Abs, Back & Neck	A. 1x5 Sit Up #59
	and/or
	B. 1x5 Leg Raise (in a chair) #60
	C. 1x5 Neck Rotation (in a chair) #1
	D. Bent Over #122
	(hold 10-15 seconds)
Light Stretch	
(20 sec. for each)	A. Side Bend 1 (in a chair) #165
	B. Torso Bend #167
	C. Full Body #169
	D. Wrist Extensor/Flexor #154

CREATE YOUR OWN PROGRAM

All of the sample programs provided in the previous section are examples of what you can create using the exercises covered within this guide. Although they are not exhaustive they do provide a broad range to help keep you challenged physically while providing variety and maintaining interest. This is crucial for any program.

You should now be able to develop your own program to meet your personal fitness goals in terms of upper and lower body resistance training, cardio, core, and flexibility/balance. Depending on your area of focus and development you may want to create one or even a group of programs to help you realize your individual goals. This section will help guide you to apply the exercises and drills I have described to create your own program.

If you do choose to create your own personal program I encourage you to build enough diversity into it to ensure a "full body workout". I also suggest that you include enough variety in your program so that your body is continually challenged in an effort to increase overall fitness.

PROGRAM DEVELOPMENT SUMMARY

The following is a brief summary of key points to consider when you create your own exercise program.

1. If you are a beginner with a lower fitness level, 20-30 minutes may be sufficient as a starting point for the first 4-6 weeks. Try to build a program that includes a warm up, cardio and resistance exercises, stretching, abs, and a cool down. If you feel your level of fitness is intermediate to reasonably advanced design a program that will provide you with a workout that is approximately 45-60 minutes in duration to start.

2. In terms of resistance training, I recommend that you begin with the larger and more complex muscle groups, like the legs and shoulders, and move to the smaller muscle groups like the biceps, triceps, and calves. You should finish your resistance workout with the abs. Keep in mind that starting with the abs periodically is a good way to mix up your workout and "shock" the body to challenge it.

3. Perform your program 2-3 times per week (ideally every other day to allow the body some recovery time) if you are at the beginner level. If you are at the intermediate to advanced fitness level, 4-6 times a week is recommended.

4. Start your program with a Warm Up (3-10 minutes) consisting of various activities and exercises to prepare and warm the body for a physically demanding workout. If you prefer to perform stretching prior to exercising, this would be the time to do so because the body is now warmed up. I recommend staying with the suggestions provided in the Warm Up as they are focused on preparing the body for the movements that will be done during your workout.

5. Add a Cardio component to the program following the Warm Up (once in a while you may want to do resistance training before cardio to add variety and test the body). For beginner fitness levels you might start with 10 minutes and work up from there. Intermediate and advance fitness levels might start at 20-40+ minutes. The cardio could include running on the spot or just running (treadmill or outside), running stairs (indoors or outdoors), cycling or any combination of the three.

   The objective is to maintain a heart rate that is compatible with your fitness level and the intensity of the workout you want to perform in order to challenge yourself and your body. A heart rate that is too low does not help cardio development while one that is too high may be harmful to your health. Include 2-4 cardio type drills.

6. In terms of Plyometrics, I strongly recommend you incorporate these types of exercises into your program only after you have reached a higher level of fitness like intermediate or advance.

7. Now add Resistance Training. This part of the program should last approximately 10-15 minutes for beginners and approximately 25-30 minutes for intermediate to advanced fitness levels. Beginners should include 2-3 exercises for each area of the body including the upper, the lower and abs. Just a reminder that when you are working the abs try to maintain a tight core (stomach) while performing the exercises as this will help with development. Intermediate and advanced training may include as many as 10-20 exercises and drills, depending on your degree of fitness and what your focus is.

   The beginner could consider performing 1 set of 5–10 exercises with 8-15 reps for each. Exercises selected will vary depending on the area of focus. The intermediate to advanced would add more exercises and drills and increase the number of sets performed for each, for example 2 – 4, depending on fitness level.

8. The last component of each session should include stretching the body after it is tired and quite warm. This is the best time to improve flexibility. Stretching will also help with cardio and resistance development while serving as a good cool down from a strenuous workout. Remember to practice breathing techniques, previously covered, to assist with the cool down. This part of the workout should typically be 10-20 minutes in duration (but could be longer) and can include some exercises to practice balance.

   The length of time dedicated to stretching depends on the intensity and duration of the workout. I recommend that you select a reasonable number of stretches that will cover all the parts of your body that you included in your workout that day. Each stretch should be performed for at least 20-30 seconds. Stretching should only be performed to a level of discomfort and not to the point where you are feeling pain. An indication of a good stretch is increased relaxation and comfort when you are done.

   As you grow older your flexibility becomes more important in sustaining your health and well being. Furthermore, it is important to remain as flexible as possible when participating in any fitness program or sport, to help prevent injuries.

Finally, you should review your fitness program and change it periodically. Remember that the primary objective is to continually challenge your body and its capabilities as it climbs to new levels of progress.

EXERCISE QUICK REFERENCE CHECKLIST

The following are some additional tips to help you get the most out of your fitness program and your workout:

1. Ensure you are properly hydrated even before starting your workout. Review the information provided earlier in this guide.

2. Always start a workout with a Warm Up (3-5 minutes) consisting of various activities and exercises to prepare and warm the body for a physically demanding workout. Try mixing it up periodically.

3. Maintain a steady intake of water during your workout with sips of water in between exercises and drills.

4. Don't forget to have short rests between exercises and drills (depending on what you are doing, the rest time can vary depending on the length and intensity of your workout). As an example, if it took you 20 seconds to complete 10 push ups, you might rest for 20 seconds before performing another set of 10. You may reduce this time if you are looking to push yourself harder. The same logic would apply to a running drill. More advanced or fit individuals may avoid rest to increase the level of cardio intensity even within the resistance component of the workout. This would be especially true if you are doing some turbulence training that includes an exercise for "active rest" where effectively, there is no idle rest involved.

5. Don't forget to breathe while you are performing various exercises and drills. Although some feel that you should exhale while increasing tension, and inhale while releasing, the main thing is that you at least continue to breathe through an exercise.

6. I suggest that initially exercises be performed in the same order as they appear in this guide. As your comfort level with the exercises improves (4 – 6 weeks) you may consider shifting them around.

7. Depending on your comfort level you can start with higher or lower reps for each exercise. What I have provided is simply a guide. Everyone will start at a different level based on their own personal fitness. Select what works best for you.

8. Pay attention to your count and form when executing drills and/or exercises. Typically, for the resistance training that uses body weight, a 2 or 3 count is appropriate to deploy increased resistance to a muscle and realize the full benefit of the exercise.

9. Don't forget to stretch correctly after each workout! Facilitate a Cool Down during the stretching period by practicing slow breathing (pranayama) techniques to assist with recovery. Initially try breathing "in" to a count of 3 and "out" to a count of 3. Over time you might try a count of 5. Proper breathing along with body stretching will help to remove lactic acid from the body and lead to a quicker recovery, improving future muscle response.

10. Consider adding 1-2 reps for each resistance exercise each week and adding 5-10 seconds to cardio drills each week. Once reps and/or time have been doubled go back to the original set of reps and time but double the sets. For example, lunges would change from 24 reps each leg to 2 sets of 12 for each leg. Start the entire cycle again by adding reps and time to each exercise or drill each week.

11. Economy of effort does not work. Don't be afraid to put effort into your workouts and you'll be pleased with the results. It is healthy to sweat!

HEALTHY EATING SUGGESTIONS

No fitness program will be completely successful unless it has a nutritional component with it. Although nutrition is a very personal choice it is critical to overall health and fitness. There is enough information within this guide to create awareness towards a healthier lifestyle that will support the increased physical demands of your fitness program.

One of the greatest challenges associated with eating properly is to stay with a nutritious approach as a way of life. Certainly if you can maintain healthier eating habits with your partner, and your family, it does become easier. There is nothing more difficult than to try to maintain a nutritious meal program when your household is constantly filled with less healthy food.

It is also much easier for children to follow the lead of their parents if they are seen eating nutritiously. Parents do need to "walk the talk" to help their children with a healthy lifestyle so they may avoid future health challenges. Keep in mind that the key to a healthy diet is to eat a variety of foods.

One of the main rules of healthy eating is that you should try to eat every 2 or 3 hours. By doing this, you won't go hungry and your metabolism runs higher all day. If you have the right mix of food, you won't experience those horrible "hit the wall" feelings that leave you reaching for caffeine or some chocolate.

Dinner should be your lightest meal of the day. It doesn't make sense to fill yourself up with calories that you won't burn off after dinner. Instead, consume food such as complex carbs, like rice and starches, at the beginning of the day when you are more likely to be the busiest and have a better chance of burning the calories away.

You may have experienced that "hit the wall" feeling in the middle of the afternoon. Some people experience it mid-morning as well. Typically, this feeling is due to falling blood sugar and/or unstable insulin levels. As a result, you may experience feelings of dizziness, sweating, or sleepiness. When you feel these symptoms, you should try to eat a combination of complex carbohydrates and lean proteins, for example cottage cheese with fruit or an apple with a tablespoon of nut butter (does not have to be peanut butter).

When these are eaten together, carbs and lean proteins offset unstable blood and insulin levels by prolonging digestion and slowing the release of sugar into the bloodstream. The goal is to maintain steady blood sugar and insulin levels. You should always try to pair complex carbs with protein. This will slow the carb to fat conversion process.

What is a proper portion size? When you make a commitment to start eating more nutritiously, you may want to measure foods until you get a feel for appropriate portion sizes. A 5 or 6 oz. portion of lean protein is about the size of the palm of your hand. This is adequate for an adult. However, children typically require more. Children have a higher metabolism, are usually more active and their bodies are still developing. Research suggests that a reasonable portion of a complex carb, involving fruits or vegetables, is a heaping handful while a serving of complex carbs from whole grains or starches is the size of a tennis ball.

GENERAL GUIDELINES

1. Try to eat 5 or 6 small meals every day which means eating about every 2-3 hours.

2. Combine lean protein and complex carbs at every meal.

3. Drink at least 2 liters, or 8 cups, of water each day. It's easier to drink 500ml of water with your meals to ensure you are adequately hydrated.

4. Try not to miss any meals, most importantly breakfast.

5. Carry a cooler type lunch bag that you can keep nutritious foods in for the day.

6. Avoid over processed refined foods. This would include foods made with anything white like white sugar and white flour.

7. Try to avoid saturated and trans fats.

8. Avoid colas and alcohol as they have high sugar content.

9. Avoid calorie laden foods like donuts, chocolate bars and potato chips (high in sodium).

10. Try to consume lots of fresh fruits and vegetables for fiber, vitamins and enzymes. Eat lots of color. Refer to government publications for recommended servings per day.

11. Try to maintain proper portion sizes.

EXAMPLE OF A TYPICAL DAY MEAL PLAN - ADULT

The following is an example of a typical day of eating for an adult with associated timeframes and food ideas. Again, this may be challenging to adopt at first but if you stay with it you will be very pleased with your results.

7:00 A.M. 1 cup cooked oatmeal topped with 1 tablespoon of ground flaxseed, bee pollen and ½ tsp. cinnamon
1/4 cup fresh berries
4 egg whites (boiled or scrambled)
1 cup of green tea
1 liter of water

9:30 A.M. 5 oz. of grilled chicken breast
1/2 medium sweet potato
500 ml water

NOON Romaine lettuce; cucumbers, tomatoes, red bell peppers with a dash of lemon juice
4 oz. baked or grilled talapia
1 cup green tea
500 ml water

2:30 P.M. 1 scoop protein powder with 1 cup water
1/2 cup raw veggies
500 ml water

5-6:00 P.M. 1/2 baked sweet potato
1 cup steamed vegetables
5 oz. grilled salmon
1 cup green tea
500 ml water

LAST MEAL 1/2 cup low fat yogurt with ½ cup diced mango
(if needed) 500 ml water and/or clear herbal tea

OTHER THOUGHTS FOR CONSIDERATION

Some hints for waking up your body:
1. as soon as you wake up, drink 500 ml of water
2. eat a breakfast of whole grains, fruits and vegetables and lean protein
3. eat only natural, whole foods
4. avoid greasy processed meats and sugary, calorie-laden foods

For the most important meal of the day (breakfast):
1. drinkable low-fat yogurt mixed with muesli
2. whole grain bread with one tbsp of natural nut butter (almond is best)
3. hardboiled egg whites with dry brown toast
4. oatmeal with 2 scoops of protein powder and a handful of raisins or ½ cup of egg whites in place of the protein powder
5. scrambled egg whites with veggies on whole grain bread
6. protein smoothie with fruit
7. ½ cup of high grain cereal with low-fat milk (or soy milk) and berries

For lunch:
1. whole or multi-grain high-fiber bread, pita or wrap
2. low fat hummus, mustard, salsa or horseradish
3. low fat cheese, goat cheese, low fat cream cheese
4. for moisture: use things like salsa, sliced avocado, fresh tomato, lettuce, spinach leaves, cucumbers, grated carrot or sprouts, balsamic vinegar, mustard, lemon juice
5. try whole-grain leftovers like rice, quinoa or couscous in a wrap

For Carb consumption:

1. eat more fruits and vegetables rather than breads, pasta, rice
2. eat whole grain products
3. monitor the portions of carbs that you eat
4. reduce the amount of refined carbs (anything white)

For Protein consumption:

1. eat protein from many sources like soy, chicken, beans
2. reduce the amount of red meat
3. eat protein at every meal (it doesn't have to be much)
4. monitor the portions of proteins that you eat

For Fat consumption:

1. eat essential fatty acids (EFAs) at every meal but avoid too much
2. eat a low fat diet regularly (monitor intake of saturated and trans fats)
3. avoid high fat snacks
4. prepare food with little or no fat (olive oil vs butter)

For Micronutrients:

1. drink at least 8 – 12 cups of water per day
2. choose a good multi-vitamin
3. eat lots of fruits and vegetables for vitamins and minerals

For Monitoring Your Weight:

1. be aware of portion sizes and overeating
2. don't keep trying new diet programs
3. combine physical activity with proper nutrition
4. make sure that your final meal of the day is no later than 6:00 p.m. whenever possible

If we can avoid doing the kinds of things that are listed below, it will help reduce the destruction of the nutrients we consume:

1. eating too much
2. eating while standing up
3. eating "on the run"
4. not chewing adequately before swallowing
5. eating after 6:00 p.m. and/or late into the night
6. consuming too much caffeine, alcohol, nicotine, or drugs
7. consuming too much sugar, sweetener, flour, refined and over-processed foods
8. using too many antibiotics and man-made drugs

CONCLUSION

Like any journey, you tend to learn more if you are open to new ideas, approaches and concepts. I believe the approach you take towards a health and fitness program is no different. The intent of this guide is to provide yet another piece of health and fitness information in this rapidly advancing area that has gained a lot of attention in the last few years. My hope is that this book has helped provide you with a convenient and affordable fitness option that really only requires an investment of your time and effort.

I have learned over the years that there is a greater opportunity for success, whether in business or personal life, if three ingredients are present. The first is a goal and/or vision. This is the responsibility of each individual to determine where he or she wants to go or end up. The second is having a roadmap – determine what you have to do to get there. The last involves removing the excuses as to why they can't get there. Hopefully this guide provided some assistance in creating a roadmap to pave the way for you in terms of your fitness and wellness goals.

This guide has been written and structured using my many years of health and fitness knowledge and will hopefully provide you with enough variety to sustain your interest in lifelong fitness. If you follow the physical fitness information contained in this guide, you should be in a position to maintain a healthy and fit program for your lifetime. All you need to apply is your own energy and creativity.

I recognize that each individual will progress at a different rate and this program allows for that variation of development. In some cases, this program alone may not be totally sufficient for certain individuals. However, it does provide options that can be explored to introduce cross training and other fitness disciplines in terms of a workout or formalized fitness program for any age.

This program can be a good start for adolescents, between the ages of 8-14, before weight training should even be introduced. Between the ages of 15-35 individuals may feel this program is insufficient for developing muscle growth, especially for those that are involved with various types of competitive sports. However, I still encourage its use, or various components of it, to supplement any weight training program for "cross training" and cardiovascular development.

Many professional athletes are now using programs of this type, or some aspects of it, in their off season to support their training efforts. For those that simply want to maintain or improve their present level of fitness, the fitness approaches within this guide will work for you as they continue to do so for me.

It is safe to say that you never complete a fitness program because the fitness journey never ends. It is ongoing and becomes part of your daily routine. Those that are committed to fitness and a healthy lifestyle stay with it as a regular course of life. In doing so, they are rewarded with higher levels of energy, looking and feeling better, reduced levels of stress, reduced risk of injury, and generally greater success in everything they set out to do. No different than eating, sleeping or going to work or school, a true commitment to fitness involves a daily routine with some form of physical activity to remain strong and healthy.

Even if you only use certain aspects of this guide, I am confident it will provide you with some valuable life skills that can be taken forward for your life. If you feel healthier, gain more confidence and set the stage for future physical and professional development, you have graduated to the next level. Always keep in mind that you are only really competing against yourself. If you are happy with your own progress against the goals that you set, you are succeeding!

ACKNOWLEDGEMENTS

Fitness for Your Life is the culmination of over 40 years of my physical fitness experiences and has taken time to complete. While writing this guide, a number of other associated publications have given me some ideas on presentation, content and approach so that I may more effectively present my program to my readers. I would like to recognize those authors and publications shown below.

Andes, Karen (1995). A Woman's Book of Strength, First Edition. The Berkley Publishing Group, New York.

Brown, Lee E. & Ferrigno, Vance A. (2005). Training for Speed, Agility and Quickness, 2nd Edition. Champaign, IL: Human Kinetics.

Church, M. (1997). Mastering Personal Fitness Training. Australia: Fast Books.

Clark, N. (1997). Sports Nutrition Guidebook. Champaign, IL: Human Kinetics.

Cook, B. & Stewart, G. (1996). Strength Basics: Your Guide to Resistance Training for Health and Optimal Performance. Champaign, IL: Human Kinetics.

Howley, E.T. & Franks, D. (1992). Health Fitness Instructor's Handbook. Champaign. IL: Human Kinetics.

Reno, Tosca (2007). The Eat – Clean Diet Cookbook. Robert Kennedy Publishing, Mississauga, Ontario

Personal Program Progress Track Sheet

Date: _____

Warm Up (3 - 5 min.) _____

Cardio _____

Exercise/Drill	Week 1	Week 2	Week 3	Week 4	Week 5	Week 6	Week 7	Week 8	Week 9	Week 10	Week 11	Week 12
	REPS x SETS											

Personal Program Progress Track Sheet

Date: _____

Warm Up (3 - 5 min.) _____
Cardio _____

Exercise/Drill	Week 1	Week 2	Week 3	Week 4	Week 5	Week 6	Week 7	Week 8	Week 9	Week 10	Week 11	Week 12
	REPS x SETS											

Personal Program Progress Track Sheet

Date: _____

| Warm Up (3 - 5 min.) | _____ |
| Cardio | _____ |

Exercise/Drill	Week 1	Week 2	Week 3	Week 4	Week 5	Week 6	Week 7	Week 8	Week 9	Week 10	Week 11	Week 12
REPS x SETS												